The Art of Sensual Female
DOMINANCE

The Art of Sensual Female
DOMINANCE,
A Guide for Women

CLAUDIA VARRIN

ILLUSTRATIONS BY CYNTHIA LECHAN

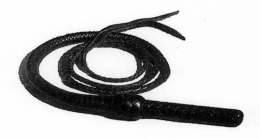

CITADEL PRESS
Kensington Publishing Corp.
www.kensingtonbooks.com

To Kevin
And With Thanks, for Their Love and Support
Ava Taurel
Franco and Renee Orobello

CITADEL PRESS BOOKS are published by

Kensington Publishing Corp.
850 Third Avenue
New York, NY 10022

All Kensington titles, imprints, and distributed lines are available at special
quantity discounts for bulk purchases for sales promotions, premiums,
fund-raising, educational, or institutional use. Special book excerpts or
customized printings can also be created to fit specific needs. For details,
write or phone the office of the Kensington special sales manager:
Kensington Publishing Corp., 850 Third Avenue, New York, NY 10022,
attn: Special Sales Department, phone 1-800-221-2647.

CITADEL PRESS and the Citadel logo are Reg. U.S. Pat. & TM Off.

First printing: 1998

20 19 18 17 16 15 14 13 12 11 10

Printed in the United States of America

Library of Congress Cataloging-in-Publication Data

Varrin, Claudia.
    The art of sensual female dominance : a guide for women / Claudia Varrin :
    illustrations by Cynthia Lechan.
        p.   cm.
    "A Citadel Press book."
    Includes bibliographical references and index.
    ISBN 0-8065-2089-2
    1. Sexual dominance and submission.   2. Sex instruction for women.   3. Sex
    (Psychology)   I. Title.
HQ79.V37   1998   97-45544
613.9'6'082—dc21   CIP
ISBN 0-8065-2089-2

Contents

Disclaimer

This book explores controversial and risky sexual activities. Neither the author of this book nor its publishers assume any responsibility for the exercise or misuse of the practices described in this book.

As the cautions in the book make clear, D&Sers are keenly aware of the danger inherent in what they do and take all care and precautions to reduce risk, anticipate problems, understand them when they happen—and most important—to avoid them. The author has provided only basic health warnings in the appropriate chapters to remind the readers of the risks involved.

D&Sers make a real and explicit distinction between consensual acts between adults for mutual pleasure and any and all acts of violence against nonconsenting partners. Imposing any sexual activity on a reluctant partner is immoral and offensive. Imposing it on an unwilling partner is a criminal offense. Additionally, the law varies from state to state. In some jurisdictions, these activities are illegal even between consenting partners.

Preface

If you are reading my words curled up in your favorite chair, looking for a little titillation and some ideas to put a flame back in your love life, then one thing is for certain. You have chosen to read about Dominance and Submission (D&S) because you already have a lively, and positive, interest in it.

Two questions may have popped into your mind when you first picked up this book. What makes straight, or "vanilla" sex as D&Sers call it, so different from the techniques, in particular sensual female domination, that you will be introduced to here? And can you "master" (or "mistress" if you prefer) those techniques and harness the powerful vamp/bitch/love goddess inside you? I will answer both questions as fully and sincerely as possible, because it is important to me that you understand the emotional and sexual fulfillment and joy that dominant/submissive sex has brought to my life. Besides, whether you're a "top" or a "bottom," D&S is romantic and fun!

Why the sudden interest in D&S, a practice that has been in the closet for centuries? Why is D&S now surfacing as a mainstream lifestyle, or lovestyle as I call it? That it's exciting, erotic, and empowering are the first reasons. That it's an escape from boredom is another. Maybe things are getting a little dull, a little humdrum? Has twice a week become standard in your bedroom? You can tell me; I know, I've been there. Does he still have the "not-tonight-honey" blues, even though it's been over a week! Besides, look around! What do you see? Machines! Faxes, modems, keyboards, and screens. Wouldn't leather and lace and high heels look deliciously wicked? Wouldn't candles be nicer, cozier, sexier than a halogen floor lamp? What sounds surround us nowadays? Beeps and bloops, blips and buzzers! What happened to the low-pitched, sultry voice that sent a frisson down a man's spine? *Press one if you have a touch tone phone . . .* How about wielding a sexy black riding crop as a symbol of your authority instead of a mouse? A *mouse*, for God's sake! Shouldn't someone be shrieking, "Eek!"? Where did the fun, the excitement go? What happened to our sense of adventure? What happened to our romantic natures? When was the last time you quivered with passion? We have forgotten the power of a lover's words because most of us don't hear them anymore. But "living dangerously" truly *is* dangerous in the real world these days, so let's be dangerous types in the safety of our bedrooms. I'm going to turn you into a deadly weapon, sister!

Indulge me, please. I love to talk about D&S. So, before I answer those burning questions, I'd like to tell you why I embraced D&S and then give you an overall picture of how D&S is seen by the people doing it these days.

I had two main reasons for becoming deeply involved in D&S. The first one is an internal well of power I had only glimpsed before and now have in my control. The second reason is something we all love: pleasure. When I was a professional, I was always and only a "top" (a dominant). And at first, I loved "topping" (dominating) the men who came to me with their secret desires and took great pleasure in acting out their desires on/with/for them. But in my private life I was and always have been submissive, even when that "private" life consisted of only fantasies. So D&S worked with the different aspects of the way I prefer to take my pleasure. I love pleasure (who doesn't?). And D&S is an exciting and exotic variety of pleasure.

Why Me?

As I have already pointed out, I am not a member of any medical profession, so what makes me qualified to write this book? Dominas aren't doctors or therapists, although many will say that they find their work therapeutic, as do their partners. One doesn't need a degree; imagination, creativity, and confidence are not college subjects. What I bring to you is S&M/D&S experience combined with a lifestyle and values that are very similar to your own. A real person just like you, who worries about the bills and that extra ten pounds and the spot on her favorite dress. Only my dress happens to be made of leather!

Many years ago, a friend asked me if I would like to meet a woman who needed women she could train as dominatrixes. Intrigued, I said yes. The woman I met was Ava Taurel, and after a few short moments together, she decided that I possessed that undefinable quality that made me a dominant female. The day I became a professional dominatrix was liberating. One delightful but unexpected side effect of letting my powerful dark side out of the closet was the freedom of expression it lent the rest of my life. Suddenly I was in a world where the men outnumbered the women eight to one, and I was able to pick and choose who I wanted to grace with my presence. Life had become interesting again. My self-esteem skyrocketed. Men's heads turned when I walked by them with a new variety of assurance that proclaimed *I was different.*

My juices once again started to flow, especially the sexual and creative ones. I plunged into the D&S life, being a guest panelist on five different talk shows promoting the benefits of D&S sex. I spoke to magazine writers and newspaper people. Several college students approached me about being their "final" exam, and I was delighted to write and appear in their videos. One class was polled before the video was shown; less than half had a positive interest in D&S. But polled again after the video, several students came away with a new, enlightened opinion on D&S and its practitioners.

Long before any of that happened, Ava trained me in safe domination. She explained to me that there were two kinds of dominants: active and passive. Rather than bore you with a long, lingo-loaded explanation of the terms, let me just put it this way. An "active" top is very hands-on, very assertive in everyday life, like Ava herself. If you don't move fast enough, she has the size and strength to move you to her liking. I, alternatively, am a passive dom: I give a command and I simply expect it to be obeyed. But active or passive, she agreed to give me the necessary training. Since I already knew how to handle a flogger, or whip, the first lesson she gave me was an anatomy lesson on one of her slaves. (You'll find anatomy lessons in both the "Discipline" and "Foot Fetishes" chapters.)

From there, we progressed to spanking lessons, paddling lessons, and caning lessons, all on different slaves who volunteered for the purpose. As part of each lesson on corporal punishment, the slave, or submissive, would describe to Ava how the beating I gave them felt and rate my abilities. Of course, any form of corporal punishment makes noise, and you can tell if the beating is a good one based on the sound of it. Instruction was given in bondage: body and cock and ball; safety tips were passed on. Ava described to me what I could say to the submissive to heighten the experience for him. She explained the psychological impact the slave's submission would have on him as well as what makes a good spanking. This and much more went into my training before I could see clients.

It was during this time that Ava and I formed a lasting friendship. Nothing in my life had prepared me for her kind of person. She's totally sane, but some of her opinions are completely flipped out. She is one of the most intelligent people I have ever met and one of the dizziest. Her mind is open and inquiring and filled with dreams, yet she is almost old enough to be my mother. Her understanding and acceptance of the practice of S&M, in herself, in me, and in others, made me feel for the very first time that there was nothing wrong with being sexually dominant or submissive and acting out those fantasies.

Meeting Ava was certainly not my first encounter with S&M; I have been indulging in it, if only mentally and somewhat guiltily, ever since I could remember. As a child, my fantasies were of a sadomasochistic nature; as a teen, I read everything I could find that even alluded to S&M. When I became sexually active, I was always able to find a man I could dominate in some way or one who could in some way be made to dominate me. I developed an "eye" for picking out men whom I could interest in playing. When the bottom directs the action, it is called "topping from the bottom." I didn't mind—it was better than just plain vanilla sex.

Through my friendship with Ava, I came out of the closet and into the light—the light of guilt-free sexuality, assertiveness, and confidence. I became better at expressing myself, verbally and on paper, and rekindled my high school dream of being a writer. With her support, I was able to tap into an internal well of power, sexual and nonsexual, that I had only glimpsed or suspected before. By becoming a professional dominatrix, I was able to focus on this well and harness its power for use in my everyday life. The harnessing of this new wealth of internal power emitted a powerful aura, a shine, that I didn't feel I was projecting before.

What is this aura and what's in it for you? Since each of us has this internal well of power, why not tap into your well on demand and have a little fun with it? Once you discover this well of power you will find that others notice it too. To them, the well might manifest itself as confidence, intelligence, and animal sexuality. Maybe you will walk a little taller or strut a little better or slink a little more sinuously than before. Who knows? But this aura will project itself even when you are not aware you are projecting it.

When I freed my sexuality from its self-induced and societal bonds by being dominant, it helped me to take control of my life and keep it. And I was certainly happier for it. I found a new authority inside of myself (I think it was always there, in a fantasy) and brought it forth, exhibiting dominant behavior at home, initially in little ways—a "new" sharing of household chores followed up by a rigorous enforcement of the new division of duties. In dealing with the rest of the world, I learned that unpleasant men are just little boys in men's clothes and that these men needed to be disciplined. Disorganized men needed to be whipped into some semblance of order. Late men needed to be taught a lesson in timekeeping. And I was just the one to do it.

Great, you say. But how did I manage to tap into and harness that well? I am not a psychiatrist or a psychologist or a help-line therapist, so my answers to you are based solely on my own experiences. And, the method I used may or may not work for you. Okay, how did I manage to use my newly-found sexual dominance to gain and keep control of my life? I thought about what I did as a professional dominatrix and brought it into my everyday life. Men paid to obey me, to worship my feet, to launder my handwash, to be beaten by me and humiliated by me. They did it without question and accepted my punishments with relish. *Relish.* One even paid to lounge in my dirty bath water!

I began to speak to outsiders with the same cool but courteous authority I used with my slaves. Yes, I cared about their feelings, my dominance was not a reason for abuse, but of course they wanted to serve me, obey me, win my approval. Why shouldn't they? I never raised my voice or used foul language; it was totally unnecessary. Nor am I a brutal person. I speak in low cool tones, as if I expect, and deserve, all due respect and the best of service, no matter what that service is. I am polite but firm, courteous but in charge, and my tone of voice, although melodious and pleasant, also tells the listener I will brook no BS. I act as if everyone is absolutely delighted to go that extra step for me, to make that call to see if the other store has those shoes in my size, to push my grocery cart to my car and unload it into my trunk! They believe in my power because it is so apparent that I believe it. This aura and a confident smile has men giving me their seats on the bus, holding the door for me, even letting me in front of them in line.

Okay, fair enough, you are not going to become a professional dominatrix to unleash the sexually dominant voodoo inside of you. But you don't have to! All that time and training. That's what I'm here for; that's why you have this book! Been there, done that, absolutely loved it! Now it's time to share with my friends. Let them in on the fun and games.

Regarding Safe Sex. . .

Missing throughout the book are references to safe and safer sex. This is not to say that the author does not practice or believe in safe sex; mention of it has been omitted because the book is written for couples in a monogamous relationship where safe sex is not an issue. Additionally, since D&S play does not have to culminate in intercourse or oral sex, protection from disease may not be an issue.

However, for those of you not currently in a monogamous relationship, all safe, and safer, sex standards apply. First, a visual inspection of the genitals should be made. A condom, male or female, should be worn during vaginal intercourse; two during anal intercourse would be safer. A dental dam should be used for oral sex on the female; an unlubricated condom for oral sex on the male. Latex gloves, either surgical or fetish, or "finger covers" should be worn on fingers that are entering the anus or vagina. The proper water-soluble, oil-free lubricant should be used to preserve the integrity of the latex. Vaseline or oil-based lubricants should be kept away from latex as it will eat it away and the latex will rip.

The Art of Sensual Female
DOMINANCE,

~ 1 ~

Stepping Behind the Veil

I n the garden of love, romance, and eroticism, D&S can be a powerful tool. D&S play extends foreplay, builds anticipation, and embellishes sexual pleasure. For many men, a thirst for variety seems to be an integral part of their psychological makeup. A man may simply want another woman just because she is another woman. There could be nothing "wrong" with you at all—other than your inability to metamorphose yourself into someone else. If you have the raw material and someone to tell you how to use it, D&S can provide you with the technique and confidence to turn yourself into a different woman, or many different women, at will. Leather one night, lace the next, the sweet, kindly mistress who treats her slave like a pampered pet, then the stern taskmistress who doles out punishment for each infraction. The possibilities are only limited by your combined imaginations!

Personally, I prefer to use the term sadomasochistic sex, S&M, as the broad, all-compassing phrase for what we will discuss here. To me and many other D&Sers "SM" means "Sexual Magic" or "Sex Magic" because of the powerful and emotional exchanges that players can experience. But I am also very aware that labels and stereotyping are bad things and that the term sadomasochistic sex is often misunderstood. No distinction is ever made between a criminal sadist (for example, a torturer and serial-killer of women like Ted Bundy) and the sexual sadist who, with the consent and participation of the other party, engages in activities that appear painful to an outsider but are truly an erotic and romantic experience for the participants. For that reason, I will use dominance and submission, "D&S," which has become the phrase of choice to denote the many delightful sex games we play other than the giving and receiving of pain.

What is the difference between a sexual sadist and a dominant? Between a sexual masochist and a submissive? A sexual sadist, although she appears dominant because of the pain she inflicts, may not be interested in other aspects of D&S. She may not want or require any sort of service like a pedicure or the handwash; her taste is for giving pain to heighten sexual pleasure. Alternatively, a dominant may embrace a much broader spectrum of the D&S realm and engage in role-playing, gender swapping, foot worship, or any other number of pastimes, as well as use pain as an instrument of pleasure. A sexual masochist is the perfect partner for the sadist uninterested in domination. The masochist's source of pleasure lies in receiving pain, and often the masochist is uninterested in any form of servitude or submission. The submissive, however, relishes serving the mistress in any way she sees fit and that includes the acceptance of pain, either as discipline or for her pleasure. So, not all doms are sadists, not all sadists are doms, not all subs are pain sluts, and pain sluts needn't be submissives.

The catch phrase of the D&S community is "safe, sane, and consensual" and this holds true for advanced players as well as beginners, singly or as a couple. As a matter of fact, D&Sers run around spouting "safe," "sane," and "consensual" as if they were the only three words in the English language! Certainly at times one may like to gag them for this tendency, but they all say it because it is *true*. Boring but true. D&S play is a mutually agreed upon scenario involving some aspect of D&S play that both parties have participated in creating and both enjoy acting out. The scene may be simple or elaborate, physical or psychological, but both parties have had a hand in its creation, and it contains elements of sexual interest to both.

"If it's painful, you're not doing it right." The pain given and received in D&S play is not, as you have guessed, painful at all. It is not the extreme portrayed by those who have little or no true knowledge of it. The playing, while it may not appear loving to a vanilla person, is very loving indeed. In what a friend called the "dark side of our search for spirit," an extraordinary trust is developed in the D&S relationship. With a loving, caring partner the D&S relationship becomes something very special, quite extraordinary. I have experienced playtimes when I have felt a spiritual connection with my partner in a D&S relationship that I never experienced in a vanilla one. When I give him "the look" that we are about to play, his heart begins to pound in his chest with lust, and he pants in anticipation of the pleasure we will share. Knowing I know his secret heart and that I care for him, his trust in me frees him and his spirit soars to new heights of sexuality and submission. Free from guilt, he is free to continue to explore and experience the great joy his sexuality gives him. For me, each playtime with him brings new levels of fulfillment, expansion, and personal growth.

The D&S relationship is a complex one. Because of the level of trust involved and the fact that some, if not all, D&S play has some element of risk or danger in it, D&S practices are most satisfying when performed with a regular partner, as in a monogamous relationship. Over time, other couples may be invited to join or a single female or male who may be submissive to the dominant or a codominant may be brought in to play and enhance sexual pleasure. But traditional, and unsafe, one-night stands are uncommon in D&S. A one-night stand is usually a prearranged evening with a dominant known to the submissive and whom the submissive has agreed to be dominated by. The play parameters in these one-nighters are set well beforehand and are usually much stricter than with the submissive's regular dominant.

Often the D&S relationship is a mirror image of the roles the two people play in life. Life with another person is often a stream of compromises, a division of responsibilities and labor, and a series of consultations, thought-weighing, and decisions. In the real world, the assignment of life's tasks is usually doled out according to gender. The man hangs the shelves, the woman does the laundry. But what if the man is all thumbs and the woman feels unsafe alone in the basement where the laundry room is located? If this couple had the enhanced communication the D&S relationship fostered and their skills were up to it, he would be doing the laundry (or at least having it sent out) and she would be hanging the bookshelves. I know a couple who had this exact problem and they solved it by switching responsibilities: he did the grocery shopping, cooking, and the laundry; she, on the other hand, painted the house, sanded floors, and, yes, put up the bookshelves.

D&S relationships can be conducted on many levels, from the once-a-year birthday spanking to a full, lifestyle relationship. Each couple will find their middle ground when they decide how much D&S play they want to let into their lives. For some, playing two to four times a month will be all their schedules (and libido!) can accommodate. This takes planning and a plan takes time. For others, a definite once-a-week session plus little tidbits thrown in during vanilla sex will hardly suffice. Once having had a taste of a D&S relationship with its enhanced sexuality, open communication, and guilt-free fantasies, it is hard to imagine going back to straight old vanilla sex. D&S sex casually introduced into a relationship for spice but not total lifestyle is like a sharp sauce. You may not want it on your meat and potatoes every night but once in a while it is very enjoyable.

The most difficult part of any relationship is getting one partner to open up and talk to the other. In a D&S communication, because of the nature of the "secrets" themselves, sharing of the secrets becomes integral to the relationship. Kind of like "this will be our little secret, our little fantasy, and the world needn't know about it." In some cases the sharing seems more like "confessing"; verbalizing one's most secret fantasies with another is often a leap of faith, and many men are not willing to take that leap. In many studies on D&S the institute or researcher has asked ordinary people like you and me and our partners to submit their fantasies for consideration. The overwhelming majority of fantasies submitted by the men had some aspect of female domination in them! The fantasies ranged from the soft, sensual surrendering of control to a beautiful and kind mistress to visions of uniform-clad amazons wielding power over life or death.

I have fantasized about S&M sex when the man I was with wasn't interested that evening, or in the rare case, not at all. Then I would have a whole S&M movie running in my mind the entire time. I have often wondered how many times the two halves of a vanilla couple have fantasized about S&M sex during straight sex unbeknownst to the other, each too embarrassed to say anything. The desire to be dominated is in many men, but communicating that desire is where they have difficulty. Imagine the level of trust he must have in you to tell you of his desire to be put in bondage, whipped for sexual pleasure, or to worship your feet. So listen to him, support him, and keep up your end of the deal by being the best top to him you can be.

Some men have told me that they fear sharing D&S fantasies of being submissive to their wife, because it would upset the balance of their authority in the home. D&S is "playtime," and the freeing and enactment of sexual fantasies is meant to enhance your relationship, not twist it. D&S is not abuse; it is loving and consensual and planned for the pleasure of both parties. The mutual delight in planning out an enactment of sexual fantasies, both yours and his, should inspire a deeper trust between you. The D&S relationship should help bring you and your partner closer together. To make D&S work, you must communicate well. If you can share intimate sexual secrets, this new openness will enhance your trust in each other that will carry over into the nonsexual parts of your lives. If you can tell him you want to spank his bottom, and not just as part of an exuberant shagging but as a planned scenario, you can tell him plenty of other things, too. At the proper time, of course.

The Questions, Please

Now let's talk about your first question: How is the variety of sex I am advocating here, sadomasochistic sex, or D&S, different from vanilla sex? Other than the accoutrements D&Sers use in their fun and games, I would have to say, not much. Wouldn't you agree that sex is in the mind? D&S sex is sex, isn't it? What I mean is that when I think back on all the hours into days into weeks into months I have spent indulging in my preference, the foremost difference that comes to mind is the three P's: Prior Proper Planning. Planning may be the fourth word in the D&Sers' vocabulary. Planning, everyone will agree, first takes place in the mind. Just like sex. (But you knew that.)

The difference is that with a *plan*, as in a D&S fantasy scenario, your sex play is no longer high-spirited shagging with a few spanks thrown in willy-nilly, but is more like a screenplay or short story with a beginning, a middle, and an ending. You, with the help of your partner, will be writing the script.

Planning is a funny thing. Some dominants, or dominas (which is another affectionate but respectful title for the female top), plan and plan and plan to the minutest detail. Absolutely nothing is left to chance. But chance still occurs. A sneezing fit is definitely a mood-breaker but how can it be prevented? If you are so planned out that a sneeze knocks you for a loop, perhaps a loose plan is better. I am a loose planner (and a sneezer) myself. But loose or tight, a plan is a plan and you must have one. You are supposed to be in charge here. (There's more on how to plan and how to write the script for your first scene in "Now What Do I Do With Him?")

Planning, as I've found by experience, makes the essential difference. And planning requires communication. Are you a good, sympathetic, nonjudgmental listener? Are you creative and imaginative? Do you consider yourself to be a good actress? And a good director? Are you good at making your thoughts and desires clear? Can you keep a straight face no matter how humorous his fantasy may seem to you? These are good qualities for D&S play (or anything else for that matter) whether you are playing the dominant or the submissive. The answers to these questions may also help you to decide if playing the domina is for you.

Now I'd like to answer your second question: Will you be able to dominate your mate? Unless he balks at the idea or you can't seem to hit upon a scenario that appeals to him, I don't see any reason why you shouldn't be able to engage in a little titillating D&S, or role-playing or bondage. "Oh, but I feel I am the submissive," you may say. Or, "I don't think I could *really* hurt him, I love him," you protest. Well, I'll let you in on a secret, or a few secrets, about being a "top" or a dominant. Everyone in the "scene" (the "scene" is what the D&S players call their lovestyle) knows that all the best tops were once bottoms! If you are not sure you can pull off the dominant role with any degree of success, there are questions throughout this introduction that will help you decide. Then if you still feel the dominant role isn't for you, you can use this book as a guide to setting up the fantasy scenes with you in the submissive role.

To make things easy, I have assumed for the sake of this book that you, the woman, *will* be the dominant and that your male partner will be the submissive. Being submissive is a state of mind, not a gender or sex-specific thing, and most people can adopt a submissive pose or stance temporarily, regardless of their sex. The art of domination, with its requisite skills and responsibilities, is a subject that requires education and guidance. Since the men we are dealing with were taught to be dominant almost from birth, it is we women who need to know how to turn the tables and sexually dominate them. The basic rules, necessary skills, and emotional outlook for domination are pretty much the same whether you are a female or male top. So all tops are "she," and all bottoms are "he."

Top or bottom, you now know that D&S isn't about pain; it's about control and it's about power. Who's had it, who's given it up, and who's got it now. D&Sers love the dynamics of the power exchange. Power is an important part of D&S play, and I don't mean just the power your partner has given to you to dominate him. I think power in itself is sexy. For the dominant, the illusion of power is thrilling. For the submissive, the illusion of powerlessness is undeniably sexy. Some men submit willingly; others put up a bit of a fight. If he fights it could be because he is unsure about surrendering control or he enjoys provoking you so you can punish him. The exchange of power for those involved with casual D&S is a game that is played for a certain length of time. Although the experience is real, the fact that the exchange is not real, or only temporary, makes the game erotically stimulating.

Along with power come limits. Both yours and his, which are to be respected. If he does not wish to be marked, then it is your responsibility to see to it that the marks do not last for more than a few minutes. But you can test and push and stretch his limits as time passes and you become more secure in your knowledge of each other, and constantly enhance the D&S experience.

The Glitterati, Fetterati, and Perverati

Who, you may ask, plays D&S games? D&Sers come in all shapes, sizes, ages, persuasions, and occupations. Doctors, lawyers, judges, computer programmers, dancers, teachers, small and large business owners, butchers, bakers, candlestick makers—any one or all of them could practice or fantasize about D&S. Many have advanced degrees in everything from the arts to nuclear physics. But, as in all things that take some skill and/or some amount of instruction, there is one level you enter at and other levels to which you progress.

Terms for these levels of interest differ from place to place. My personal favorites for these levels are the Glitterati, the Fetterati and the Perverati. Coined by Kevin McCain of London, these three terms neatly describe the dressed-for-it set, or posers; the genuinely interested; and the more advanced and serious players. No stereotyping distinction is made regarding sexual preference or orientation, therefore leveling the field and sorting everyone by their level of involvement and experience. (I, your guide, rank among the Perverati.)

But who are these people?

The Glitterati are those who follow S&M as a fashion statement— the See and Be Seeners (in the old days we called them "posers"). You can see them hanging around "mixed" club parties and special events in their S&M gear, avidly watching any scene being performed by the Perverati when not dancing the shine off their PVC miniskirt or tripping over their whip. I don't mean any offense by this; before I discovered the underground scene I numbered among the Glitterati myself. Some of you may be Glitterati. It is as good a place to start as any. An interest in fetish dress could be the harbinger of a deeper interest in D&S. (And at least you have a jump on the wardrobe.)

Derived from the term "fetish," the Fetterati denotes the middle level, to which you are "promoted" when your interest expands beyond the wearing of fetish dress and lounging around in it being admired. The Fetterati dress like Glitterati and still go to the same mixed club party as Glitterati but Fetterati leave earlier. *This* is the difference, you ask? Well, to the naked eye, yes. It's what they do after they leave that makes them Fetterati. These tops may lead bottoms around on leashes and a foot scene may be glimpsed here and there, but the Fetterati are not the entertainers of D&S. They use the party as foreplay, not as the main event as do the Glitterati. The Fetterati watch the scene as avidly as the Glitterati but the Fetterati watch to learn as well as be titillated. The

Glitterati stay until closing; the Fetterati slip out early to go home and get in a few good hours of D&S play before the sun comes up!

And lastly, there are the Perverati. The Perverati are the players conducting the scenes the Glitterati and Fetterati are so avidly watching. The Perverati can dress any way they like but they usually dress like Fetterati. (Fetish dress establishes their group identity.) Even in jeans, Perverati never fail to have some piece of S&M accoutrement on them, be it a latex cock whip hanging from a key chain or a bit of string coiled up in a purse or pocket for some quick bondage. If you want to learn spiderweb bondage or mummification, the Perverati (who often cluster in dark corners and, no offense meant, groups like the Janus and Eulenspiegel societies) are the people to see. If the person you ask doesn't know what you want to know, she knows someone who knows someone who does and would be happy to set up a demonstration. How would next Tuesday be? The Perverati are driven by their sexuality. Many Perverati couples are so advanced that they no longer discuss their scenarios beforehand and have dispensed with safe words since they know each other's wants and limits so well as to make this unnecessary. This is D&S nirvana.

Then there are the Fetishists, technically classified as Perverati, and the multitudinous ways that they express their fetishes. Their fetish may be as simple as a love of leather, and they can indulge their fetish easily and discreetly in their everyday life: clothes, furniture, and/or interior of their car. Or it can be as elaborate as latex bondage. A foot or shoe fetishist may sneak sniffs and the occasional surreptitious orgasm over the shoe when the lady of the house isn't in. A simple definition of a fetishist is one who has a sexual fixation on a nonsexual object or body part.

The Fetterati or Perverati player may have an entire room in their home, or the entire basement in some cases, devoted to their play. For some, the trappings of a dungeon are essential; the mirrors and matte black walls, a leather encased bondage bench, a stockade, a hydraulic lift to stretch and suspend. To others, the dungeon happens in their minds; it is verbal domination and the presence of the mistress that thrills them and the actual physical setting is unimportant. In yet other fantasies, for example, cross-dressing or foot worship, a dungeon may not be necessary or appropriate. Cross-dressing men rent hotel rooms to smoke cigars and read the *Wall Street Journal* in lacy lingerie and marabou-toed mules. D&Sers have been known to go to great lengths to indulge their fantasies.

In this book, areas that I think fall into the realm or domain of the Perverati are noted as such. None of these things should be undertaken without guidance or tutelage and direct supervision from more experienced players.

On Being Dominant

D&S is also called "sensual domination," or "sensual female (or feminine) domination." As a sexually dominant woman, you will enjoy a position of power which may include giving your partner orders (even silly ones like "bring me an iced fruit juice"), training him ("I like my foot massaged firmly," or, "a little to the left, you're missing the spot"), putting him in bondage (what we tops call "parking him" and a good way to keep him out of your hair while you do your nails) and/or giving him pain (such a nice release of pent-up frustrations).

But being the dominant partner does not mean that you are free to do anything you want to your slave unless he has told you so himself. (And what is the likelihood of that? This is his first time.) It is a position of responsibility. Some slaves will take anything the mistress dishes out; others are very specific in their wants and desires. To put it another way, when you say, "No, I don't like that," you don't expect it to be forced on you simply because someone else says so. Real-life respect has a place here. A slave is not really that; he is not chattel or property even though you may, in the context of the fantasy, "own" him. Just as you would expect someone to respect your personal desires, you should accord that same respect and consideration to your slave. Being the dominant means that first you are in control of yourself.

The ideal femme fatale domina *can* control her slave because she obviously is in control of herself. She listens to her slave, is his mentor and guide and muse. She understands the fear and eroticism the submissive feels during play. The domina always knows fantasy from reality and provides support for her slave. She is enough of a sadist to inflict pain and loving enough to use it only as an instrument to increase pleasure. She is imaginative and creative, and cares for the emotional and physical well-being of her slave. She knows that his submission to her is a gift and that his surrender is voluntary. She knows that she has only the illusion of power and is in control with the permission of the submissive. She knows that part of being dominant means pleasing her submissive and in that sense, she is submissive to the will of the other. She respects his limits and appreciates the depth of trust he has placed in her and knows that respecting his limits is the basis for trust. She knows that D&S is not to be done in anger but that it is a creative transformation of everyday frustrations and anger into erotic play or domination.

As the dominant, you will start to develop an emotional bond with your submissive partner, born in the trust you have established in opening up about your D&S fantasies. For the length of the "play period," you will enjoy the power and dependency of your partner who has entrusted you with his secrets. This is a chance for you to go on a ninety-minute ego trip and let your imagination (and his desires) be your guide. Perhaps a little erotic coercion will help him realize that now you hold the key to his pleasure.

As a dominant woman, you will probably exhibit independent behavior that will exhilarate you and will be noticeable to those around you. Especially to your less-empowered sisters and to those men who are attracted to your power! The sexually dominant woman does not engage in the codependent behavior that so many of her sisters seem to be mired in. By tapping into her own inner well of power, she finds her strengths and "exploits" them herself. She feels complete as a person when she is alone and enhanced and complemented by her partner, not needy or reliant upon him. She doesn't walk around being apologetic for her personal power, but that doesn't mean she is rude or offensive. Playing the mistress can help you in all areas of your life because it helps you take control and stay in control. She has a firm grip on the reins of her world and makes the rules in her environment. Now picture yourself being able to consciously direct this aura to encompass the people around you. It will cloak you in mystery, and who doesn't love a good mystery?

On Being Submissive

D&S can be an act of liberation, or even a declaration of liberty, for the submissive. In some, the need to serve or surrender is deep and meaningful and D&S fulfills that need on an erotic or romantic level. For the shy, submission can be a place in time and space and mind where the introverted can shed the chains of daily or social life and soar above the clouds. In submission, he can choose to be whoever he wants and that is usually the opposite of who he is in his regular life. The dominant protects him as he explores his fantasies in a safe "sub space." D&S is a power exchange between the female and male: he submits his will to that of the domina's and she takes over the reins of control.

What does this do? It frees the submissive from feelings of guilt over his sexuality or sexual desires, and removing guilt removes a major stumbling block on the road to heightened sexuality. Many submissive fantasies are exciting specifically because they break some taboo or rule or another. Relieving him of responsibility for his actions or sexuality will allow him to let go of his inhibitions and abandon himself to the lascivious luxury of his fantasies. He needn't think, or look after himself; his mind is free to go where his mistress takes it. But first he has to want you to take control. How does one accomplish this? Communication and trust. In speaking to you of his submissive desires or fantasies, he is baring his soul. He may be telling you things that he has never spoken aloud to another person, and your acceptance of his secret desires is extremely important. Please treat this like the precious gift it is and be prepared to swallow your tongue before you laugh at what he says. Listen to him carefully and try your best to create the fantasy he shared with you. He needs encouragement and support, care and attention.

If he is interested in being a submissive, and is not a masochist per se, some questions you may want to ask him are: What does he think his main turn-on will be? Bondage? Servitude? Foot worship? Is there anything he is really afraid of? Being blindfolded? Being tied up? If he was emotionally, physically, or sexually abused as a child, does he have any "quirks" relating to that? What should you steer clear of if he does? A trigger word? Is he claustrophobic? How does he feel about closets? (Don't laugh.) Submission is the ultimate nakedness: both his clothes and inhibitions are stripped away, leaving him safely powerless. Since both of you want to do this and each knows beforehand what will be considered fun for the other, the pleasure will be mutual.

Talk to Me

The discussion of one's dominant and submissive desires is actually the most difficult part of playing at D&S. It is hard to tell someone, especially a loved one, your deepest, darkest sexual secrets. The fear of rejection or ridicule can make the most aggressive, argumentative person hesitant to voice their preferences.

Now imagine that your loving mate has mustered up all his courage and comes to you and tells you he is really turned on by your toes. Face it, ladies, this is a harmless fetish and one you can turn to your advantage. Think of all the pretty new shoes he will buy you to decorate your exquisite and delicious feet! And you, instead of saying, "I've never done it before but I'm willing to try it with you if you'll tell what you'd like me to do," come out with this snappy retort: "What!?! Toe sucking? That's disgusting. I'm not going to do that." I ask you, do you think he's going to share another one of his fantasies with you anytime soon? Of course not—he's going to attempt to meet someone—on the "side," since he is your mate—who is more accepting of his interest. Now wouldn't you rather have him eating in than dining out?

I have four different types of fantasies and I would like to think that most people enjoy all four varieties too. On the fantasy ladder, the lowest rung is the one occupied by memory fantasies. A memory fantasy is when you recall an erotic encounter that has already happened and relive it as it occurred or embellish on it. The second rung on the ladder is composed of the fantasies we know we would like to live out. The third rung is composed of those fantasies that fall into the "maybe" category. A fantasy on this rung could include consenting to nonconsensual and public humiliation. These are fantasies that, given the right time, circumstances, mood, and company, you *may* decide would be exciting to enact.

Then there is the top and fourth rung of the ladder. These are what I call "bathtub fantasies." I call them that because I masturbate in the bathtub and that is when I have these fantasies. These fantasies are so far out that even though they are lovely to think about when you are masturbating (being alone you need greater stimulation) but you would *never* want to happen to you. These could be fantasies of rape, deep submission, or branding. If you are relating a third or fourth rung fantasy to him, or he to you, be sure you understand which type of fantasy it is before either of you try to enact it. Imagine your surprise when he comes home with a piercing, done to please the mistress, when it was actually a fourth-rung fantasy!

As a woman, it is much easier for you to express and fulfill your sexual fantasies than it is for a man. There's that grim specter of rejection again. All the more reason for you to broach the subject instead of waiting for him to bring it up. In speaking to men over the years, it has been my observation that many of them have some interest in one aspect or another of D&S and would like it if their lady also manifested an interest in it. Literature containing studies supporting my anecdotal opinion are listed in the Recommended Reading guide. But the men are leery of bringing it up because they don't know what their partner's reaction will be. They are afraid of a "worst-case scenario," i.e. she is repulsed by the thought of it and leaves, or ends, the relationship.

A young woman told me that in the ten years she has been married to her husband, she has acted out all types of fantasies with him, some of them D&S oriented, has played all different women for him and often was the one who instigated their adventures. She went on to say their marriage and lovemaking were still fresh and they were both still very much in love. I thought her approach to their lovemaking was terrific and told her. But the point is, if a woman expresses an interest in fantasy bondage, there could conceivably be a line of men down the block and around the corner, ready, willing, and eager to satisfy her desires. A man's fear of rejection could, and often does, preclude his sharing of a fantasy with his significant other.

This is because the world at large does not understand D&S and considers D&S practitioners to be weird, sick, perverted, and exceedingly strange. Yet many of you already practice some aspects of D&S and don't even know it. If you have ever put on a garter belt, hose, push-up bra and pumps, then danced around the bedroom for the enjoyment of your loved one, you have engaged in what D&S players call "role-playing." You may fancy yourself an exotic dancer or you may just be getting your mate ready for a close encounter of the best kind. And you're not weird, sick, or perverted, are you? I know I'm not.

So what I am suggesting you do is open up the topic for him. I can't tell you exactly what to say since I don't know the person you will be talking to. But there are many ways to approach him. How are you at telling stories? One night, when your head is in the crook of his shoulder and you are nesting before sleep, tell him a fantasy à la Scheherazade. If you are the top, take him captive. If he is the top, describe how you feel about being his captive. Does he like to read? Leave this book where he will be sure to see it. If you see him glance at it, in interest or curiosity, (without seeming too eager) mention how much fun some of the ideas are or how funny some of the session stories were, or how much you would like to experiment with the ideas. Mark out a favorite passage or two and offer to lend him the book. (Better yet, buy him his own copy!) I wouldn't recommend this tactic with something entitled "Crazed Whip Sluts from Hell" since it might scare him off. If he likes comics, EROS makes a fine and fun line of S&M and D&S comics for just about every taste. Or rent a fetish movie from the local video shop and watch it with him. But be careful in your selection—some are of a better quality, shall I say, than others?

Or you can resort to the time-honored method of introducing it to him gently by holding his hands over his head during your regular lovemaking while you direct the action from on top. If he moans and gets mushy and cooperative, you might have a submissive tiger by the tail. If he likes that, try tying your scarf around his eyes and see what happens. (He surely won't be able to! And watch what that does to the tiger in his pants.) If he often plants a kiss or nibbles on your toes as he gives you a foot massage, suggest that he "suck it" in a soft, sexy tone. And if he does . . . you, my dear, may have a submissive on your hands! The beauty of this method is that you never have to mention the term D&S. If he likes it as much as you do, you have not hung a label on it that may turn him off.

If the physical aspect of D&S is not what you feel would appeal to your mate, skip it for the time being and go directly to the "siren" approach. The "siren" approach relies mainly on wardrobe, allure, and imagination. If he loves the way you look in your purple bra, panties, and garter belt, put them on. If your leather teddy drives him wild, put that on. Or take him to your favorite lingerie store and let him make you a present. Then go home immediately and try it on for him while it is still fresh in his mind and he is eager to see you in it.

Back at home now, dress in your wardrobe of choice, put on your best high heels (no flats allowed), fix your hair, and touch up your make-up. Get the music going. Get the candles lit. Position him on the sofa, or in his favorite chair, and make an entrance. Slink out of the bedroom in your new lingerie. Walk your sexy walk and strut in front of him. Tease him. If he reaches out for you, don't let him "catch" you. Make him work for the pleasure of your company and later on, your affections. Act as if you are a goddess and soon he will be believing you *are* a goddess.

If you feel that playing the submissive, slave girl, pleasure toy, or love slave is more to your liking, well, that's even easier than talking to him about dominating him. You barely have to talk at all! Try donning a sexy nightie or lacy bra and thong while he is in the bathroom preparing for bed. Then pose on the bed in Position Three (see chapter 11, "Positions") and wait for him to come out. He's sure to at least ask you what you are doing. Or tie yourself to the bed and wait for him. Or how about (on a night when you know he'll be home at a specific time) timing dinner to be ready thirty minutes after he walks in, present him with a drink when he arrives, take his briefcase and lead him to his favorite chair to relax while you prepare his meal—in your best lacy black bra and thong and garter and stockings!

Now let's assume things are progressing nicely, you have opened up the subject of injecting a little spark into your love life with D&S play, and he is outright happy to go along with it. So happy that he begins to dream up scenarios and comes to you with them. Then the unthinkable happens. He presents you with a fantasy that is not all that palatable to you.

Don't despair. Discuss his fantasy carefully. There may be aspects to it that appeal to you, and some minor adjustments to the overall scenario might make it workable for both of you. If his fantasy is one of the more unusual ones, consider building up to it by sharing other fantasies that are easier for you to accept. On the other hand, what if he presents you with a fantasy that is so tame as to be totally out of the realm of what you now consider to be D&S? What if his fantasy is something as mild as being kissed by a woman, possibly in a state of undress under her raincoat, behind a statue in the local museum? Piece of cake for an "award-winning" actress like you! And since this one will go so well and he will be so encouraged by your acceptance and imagination, he will be willing and eager when you present a scenario that fulfills one of your fantasies. Again, good communication between the two of you is of the utmost importance.

Two words of caution: never, ever discuss this topic while in bed with your prospective partner. Bed is the wrong time and the wrong place for any type of sexual discussion and D&S is definitely sexual. And never play at D&S in anger. Do not use D&S as an excuse to take things out on your mate. Discussion of everyday problems belongs in the realm of the everyday world, not your fantasy D&S domain. D&S is not abuse or an excuse to batter or mistreat your mate or partner. D&S is an emotionally intense game and must sustain and nurture the needs of both partners. If it ceases to be emotionally satisfying for either one of you, discuss the situation in a restaurant or over the dinner table and decide together whether or not you will continue to play.

Please listen carefully to the cautions I explain in the chapters where they are necessary. These guidelines have been fine-tuned by experienced players over the years and are important. If and when you read other books on Dominance and Submission, you will probably be saying to yourself, these people say the same things over and over again regarding safety and other issues of well-being. Are they lacking imagination or are they plagiarizing each other? The answer is "neither." If there were ten commandments of D&S, these cautions should be considered among them. That is why we all say them. They just can't be repeated often enough because their validity is recognized by everyone playing in D&S. They are laid out here to ensure that you and your partner will have a safe playtime, both physically and emotionally, and will want to continue to experiment together.

Questions to Ask Yourself

You have already decided that you are a good communicator and a good listener but we know that isn't all that it takes to be a good mistress. Yes, yes, you are creative and imaginative and articulate. But have you ever imagined yourself to be Emma Peel? Brenda Starr? Wonder Woman? Did you admire Sarah Douglas's mad Kryptonese villainess in *Superman II*? Didn't you just drool over her wonderful black leather outfit and thigh-high boots? What about Michelle Pfeiffer as the glorious Catwoman in *Batman Returns*? I wanted that latex catsuit for myself. And someone, or several someones, worked very hard at that spit shine—you could see yourself in it! She was very good with a bullwhip, too, and very sexy.

Or did you want to be Nancy Drew, always tied, gagged, and locked in a closet somewhere, in need of rescue and a strong male figure? When you played cowboys and Indians, were you the one always asking to be tied to the tree? Did you melt when Lois Lane was rescued by Superman? If you answer with a heartfelt "yes" to these or similar questions, the submissive role is for you. Speaking for myself, if the bad guy, or girl, has on some really cool fetish wear, I'm on their side.

Not into fetish wear yourself? Prefer strong women in cotton and linen? Rather wield the pen and investment portfolio than the sword? That's actually easier than playing the bitch-goddess because there are so many more role models around. Everyone has something that can be pressed into service as wardrobe for the executive type. Even a skirt and a crisp blouse will do. If you have a business suit or coatdress, that's perfect. The men who like this type of wardrobe are intimidated by a woman in a business suit. And that means empowerment for you.

How to play the role? Think of the offices you have worked in; now remember the worst bosses you have worked for. Roll all of their bad qualities into one and there you are! Wall Street Wild Woman!

And the last, but not least, wardrobe choice is lingerie. I think every romantic woman has a place in her heart for lingerie. I have a few drawers of it myself. When all else fails, black, purple, or red lingerie with stockings and high heeled pumps will slay him every time. Slink out of the bathroom and lounge on the couch. You know how; you've done it a million times when no one is watching. Put your feet up on him and use him as a footstool. Isn't that nice, especially when your feet are cold? The real beauty of lingerie is that it doesn't limit who you can be in a role. Dressed head to toe in leather, you *are* the Leather Mistress. Lingerie allows you to be the vamp, or the bitch, or the type of mistress who pampers her pets.

Don't go for the clothes aspect? Disappointing but not a disaster. Have you ever seen a movie with a female character that you really liked? Did you ever go home and pretend that you were the one dishing it with the male lead? Can you toss back the actress's lines before she says them? My favor tossbacks are: "With, or without?" scripted for the Mona Demarkov character in *Romeo Is Bleeding* and "You know how to whistle don't you? You just put your lips together and blow," scripted for Slim (Lauren Bacall) in *To Have and Have Not*. The real point here is that playacting, being an actress, even if you are only playing the strong side of yourself, is part and parcel of domination. Are you a good actress, or feel that you could be, if given the chance? This could be it.

Still undecided about your dominant abilities? Are you aggressive during your regular lovemaking? Good. Do you like getting on top and directing the "action"? Very good. Do you consider yourself to be sexually adventurous? Oh, quite good. And passionate? Even better. Receptive to new ideas? And nonjudgmental? Excited by things that are a little taboo or dangerous? Still yes? Excellent!

By now you have answered several questions regarding how you feel about your communication skills, your latent acting abilities, your preference in wardrobe, and your abilities as a director. If most of your answers were yeses, you may already be engaging in a little clandestine D&S and this book will help you broaden your repertoire. If your answers were mostly yeses and maybes, especially in communication skills and acting and wardrobe questions, I see no reason why, with the help of this book, you cannot have a working knowledge of the D&S basics in a very short time. If your answers were mostly yeses but you are more intrigued and excited by being the receiver than the giver, perhaps the submissive role is right for you.

~ 2 ~

Entering the World of
Dominance and Submission

Now that you have decided to try your hand at being a dominatrix, there are a few things you need to get started. First and
foremost is the ability to listen to what your partner, the man
in your life who has agreed to be your "slave," is telling you about his
wants and desires. Second is an open mind about his desires. Treat his
fantasies as the gift they are and don't you dare laugh. Not even if the
sight of him with your panties on his head *slays* you. Lastly is an ability
to exercise your common sense. It is his body you will be playing with
so you should learn its "nooks and crannies" before you start. Common
sense will tell you that if he turns out to be a foot fetishist, you are not
going to be able to stand on his head the first time you play. A footbath and then a pedicure, which is thoroughly explained in the "Foot
Fetishes" chapter, is a better idea for the beginner. Go slowly at first if
your partner is new to D&S or trying it out mainly for your benefit.

The Safe Word

The very next thing you need is also something you will not have to
purchase. It is a "safe word" and everybody has had one even if certain
members of the Perverati have relinquished theirs. A safe word is what

your slave will say when things get too close to what he perceives to be his limits. A safe word will let you know for sure when "no" is really no and "stop" is really stop. Have him say his full name or pick a word that will not come up in the normal course of your play. "Red" is easy to remember as a full stop word; "yellow" stands for "slow down." However, "mercy" is the standard word for all slaves to all mistresses when in distress. "Pity" is what he can say when he wants you to slow down or lighten up so he can catch his breath. Pity means "This is going good, just take your time", or "It's going to fast for me to absorb, so slow down", or just "Slow down, I need to think about this". But any words will do: cupcake, houseplant, whatever . . .

Since your submissive is male, you may prefer to pick a word your slave will feel embarrassed saying. Why? If he is embarrassed about saying that particular word, then he will be hesitant to say it. And you can test his limits further because of his embarrassment. Again the only caution is to make sure it is not a word you will be saying at any other time during your play.

If and when your slave says that safe word, you must stop what you are doing, and I do mean *immediately*. Even if you are right in the middle of a stroke, pull back and stop it. That word means he has reached his limit. If you do not stop now, all the trust and new sexual intimacy you have built up may be damaged or destroyed. Take the time to discuss what the problem was or what went wrong so it doesn't happen again. Perhaps you can work it through together. Communication is crucial before, during, and after playtime, as the scenarios should be playful and loving for both of you.

Closet Raid

There are things that you need that are not among the goddess's gifts to women. This means you will have to go on a mission to find wardrobe and "toys" in your home. Dressing up for D&S play is great fun in itself. I often do it even when I have no one suitable to play with or simply prefer to play alone. (Several mirrors located in strategic places throughout the home are strongly recommended for this pastime.) It's deliciously decadent to slip into something sexy and empowering. Now, put on the chosen garment and look at yourself in the mirror. With your new eyes, your dominant eyes, feel yourself emitting a new sexual heat and unbounded confidence.

In fact, presenting the proper dominant image is half the battle won. If you are unsure what his preferences are, ask him. If you don't care what he prefers, wear what most appeals to you. He is your slave and should be happy you are gracing him with your divine presence no matter what you are wearing. You are the mistress, after all.

I mentioned the most common preferences before: leather and/or other fetish wear such as a leather skirt and a crisp white blouse, perhaps with a tie; the same leather skirt with a lace bra and thong and lace-topped thigh-highs; lingerie including short sexy nighties or robes, teddies and bustiers; business suits or similar man-cut attire and, of course, high-heeled boots or shoes, with pumps (because you can "dangle" them) and strappy sandals (because he can worship your foot around the straps) as clear favorites. You probably have most of those wardrobe choices in your closet already!

There are also "power colors" for D&S players and especially, for you, the mistress. I allow my choice of wardrobe to be guided by what that particular color signifies. Black, the number one power color the S&M world over, is the surest choice. Red is also a preferred color as it signifies passion and confidence. Purple, denoting royalty as well as passion, is a popular choice. And white, as the opposite of black, is quite acceptable, too. Gold, silver, bronze, or copper are also powerful because they are "metal" colors. You are free to wear pink or green or blue but I would stick to the lingerie in that case. I never understood Mistress Lisa's green outfit in the movie *Exit to Eden*. Although I know that particular shade of green symbolized true love during the Wat Tyler Rebellion in medieval England, I was unsure how it related to D&S. I kept looking at it thinking, it would be beautiful in black. Or red. Or purple.

If you are role-playing, and not just being the "mistress," an outfit appropriate to the character you will be enacting is more important than the color of the garment. What I usually do in that circumstance is to wear lingerie in one of the power colors. That way when I take my dress off to tease him when he is helplessly bound; I can tease him in an appropriately hued wardrobe.

Your leg wear is a very important part of your mistress wardrobe. If your outfit calls for hosiery, make sure it doesn't have any runs in it. Black hose should be long and sheer and jet black. Fishnets are also popular with some men because of their rough texture. Garter belts worn with stockings or thigh-highs usually win out over pantyhose. But I can see the appeal some find in pantyhose. It looks like a fine, spidery piece of bondage equipment; the seam in the panty accentuates the crack of your ass so nicely and the way the cotton panty hugs your lips! Boy-leg panty or French-cut brief inset, I can hear the pantyhose enthusiasts sighing wistfully in the background now.

Ambiance

So you have ideas about your wardrobe. Now you need to prepare your home. Think about this one. You need to create an atmosphere. If your house smells like your dinner, open the windows, turn on the fan. Ditto for cigarette smoke smell. Odors (except for the delicious odor of sex) are not conducive to anything and may well be a distraction. Even if your home has a neutral smell, try burning some incense to add an exotic touch to the surroundings.

Lighting is also very important, ladies. Soft, dim, incandescent lighting is good, candles are even better and the more, the sexier. Candlelight will add to your mystery as well as take years off your age. And if you are not burning incense, scented candles will lend a pleasant aroma as well as illuminate the room. If he is particularly graceful, try using him as a candelabra by balancing the candles recommended for waxing (see chapter 13, "Sensation") on his outstretched arms.

The next factor is one that many people (especially when a man is setting up the scene) overlook: the temperature of the room. It may feel warm enough as you stand there all dressed, maybe even in latex, the coldest fabric known to mankind, but how will it feel on the exposed flesh of a naked slave? Will he be warm enough? A shivering, chattering blue object usually makes an unsatisfactory servant. If you have a fireplace, set him to building up the fire so neither one of you will be cold. But hopefully, your dominant self in your hot sexy outfit will have him so fired up he won't notice the temperature in the room!

The next "need" is something I never go anywhere without: music. Music always sets a tone whether you are at home or at a nightclub. The type of music you select for your playtime is a very personal choice, but be guided by the eroticism of what you are about to do, be guided by the sexuality of it and pick your music appropriately. I like Middle Eastern, Indian, and certain classical music for playing, such as Peter Gabriel's appropriately named soundtrack for *The Last Temptation of Christ;* "Passion" is very atmospheric for playing. I find it has a wonderful range of highly listenable Middle Eastern songs that are sexy and mysterious and impart a foreign, exotic quality to the proceedings. I also think the music of Flesh Fetish (available by mail order only, see Appendix under "New York"), any of the three Enigma releases, trance music by Synesthesia, Attrition's *Eternity*, Delirium's *Karma* and *Syrophenikan*, and Tricky's *Maxinquay* are appropriately sexy for play sessions and are available on CD.

Other popular music choices with D&Sers include the soundtracks to the movies Francis Ford Coppola's *Dracula: Love Never Dies*, *Interview With the Vampire*, and *The Hunger*. Have you noticed no metal music, or disco or country-western songs? D&Sers don't tend to play much of that sort of thing, and I think the reason for that is the music demands too much of your attention. The loud vocals, the screaming guitars, the crashing drums, the catchy chorus. It tends to confuse the issue or else you start to sing and lose the mood. The only one who should be screaming is your slave and that should be in deliciously feigned agony. Who is in charge here anyway? You or Axl Rose? He doesn't need to be tortured by both you and speed metal!

Treasure Hunt!

Now to the accoutrement you might want to consider for your first scene. If your partner likes role-playing and asks you to be a teacher or schoolmistress or even a babysitter, formal equipment is not necessary. A wooden ruler without the metal strip on the edge or a yardstick will suffice for the first two, your bare hand will do for the third role! If you are to be the mistress, or some other incarnation of her or the goddess, I would recommend that you pick up a small whip or slender riding crop as a visible symbol of your authority. In other words, to intimidate him. If you feel a crop or whip is too intimidating or just not right for this scene, try a shoelace made of lace draped around his wrists, a chain dog collar (get one that's at least twenty-four inches long), or a leather dog collar that's at least twenty inches long. Place the collar ceremoniously around his neck when you commence playing to denote that he is now yours to command and will remain that way until his mistress removes the collar.

There are many things in your home that can be pressed into service for D&S play before you decide to invest any money in more professional equipment. I would recommend stockings or pantyhose, your scarves or his neckties for bondage or gagging; clothespins or a skirt hanger as nipple clamps; sleep mask or a scarf for sight deprivation (blindfold); a wooden spoon, spatula, ruler, or yardstick, hairbrush, sole of your shoe, a Ping-Pong or other sports paddle, or his belt for discipline; a piecrust edger or feather or ice cube for sensitizing and tickling and so on. From those examples, you should be able to dig up other household items which can be made into instruments of sensual torture!

Let me ask you a few more questions. Do you like going to adult toy stores? Do you like to browse for toys and vibrators and read the descriptions for the shapes and sizes you favor? If you said yes, great. But if you said no, you still don't have anything to worry about. An enormous selection of fine-quality accoutrements, and I mean everything from clothes to whips to suspension gear, is available through the mail or the Internet. You can even order a catalogue from which you can order more catalogues! One maker of leather goods, a submissive from New York, will come to your home if you have made previous purchases.

Although each and every catalogue or toy of an adult nature that I have ever received has come very discreetly packaged, some of you many not want to have anything of this sort delivered to your home. Still no reason to worry. Are there any hardware stores near you? How about a riding or equestrian shop? In some places they call them "tack shops." A riding crop can be purchased for less than twenty dollars from any riding outfitters shop. I got my beautiful and expensive but now broken one (on someone's unworthy butt, no less) at Kaufman's on Park Avenue South in Manhattan.

While I was in the store making my selection, an attractive young couple came in to pick up her custom-made equestrian outfit. The man didn't look small enough to be a jockey and she didn't interact with him as if he was her trainer, or some other horsey professional in her life. Then I overheard him remark with great enthusiasm that he couldn't wait to get home and "get started." Since this was at five o'clock in the afternoon, I didn't think they were talking about horses. When I inquired of the nice British salesman how many riding crops Kaufman's sold each year, he confided to me, with a wink and a nod, that they sold between fifteen and twenty thousand! I personally doubt there are that many "equestrians" in Manhattan.

Maybe the chains, or other sorts of hardware, that bind you are what do it for you. Hardware stores are great places for inexpensive S&M gear; all you have to do is shop with your D&S eyes! All types of hooks, named after the letter of the alphabet it most resembles, are available here, as are eyes hooks and O-rings and anchors to keep them in the walls or ceiling. If drilling into the frame of your house isn't your thing, the hardware store will still work for you. Chains, cut to order, can be used with a quick-open hook for those of you who are not good at tying ropes. These can be looped around and under the metal bedframe and pulled up on to the mattress to tie him hand or foot to the bed. I like to put his chains in the freezer for a few minutes just to make him suffer. I mean shiver.

I made my very first spreader bar from items purchased at the hardware store. I bought a wooden closet pole, one-inch in diameter, and had the store cut it to thirty inches for me. Then I bought those little rubber cups to put on the sawn ends to guard against splinters. I screwed eye hooks into each end; this helped to hold the cups on, too. A large eye hook was screwed into the middle in case I wanted to thread a rope through it to his collar or hand restraints. A few coats from a can of glossy black spray paint and I had a spreader bar. And no one had a clue as to what I was doing when I bought the stuff.

Handcuffs are available at local adult toy stores and through catalogues. I got my set of handcuffs, ankle cuffs, and waist and handcuff chains from a retired police officer. Rope can be purchased in regulation white at hardware stores and the new sexy black is available at marine outfitters and through catalogues. Bondage is a very popular pastime and is often indulged in, if you will, by people who are not into any other aspect of the scene. Many dominants like to be put in bondage and switch with their mates. Can you just imagine the fight over it? No, you tied me up last. Now I want to be tied up. No, me. No, ME. Personally, I love bondage.

Imaginative schemers that they are, D&Sers will plan and connive for days and shop till they drop for just the right accessory, the perfect item, for their fantasy scene. D&Sers are also a creative lot when it comes to making and finding new toys, and soon you too will develop an eye for what we of the Perverati call "pervertables."

On a practical note, I suggest you stock the fridge with beverages and snacks before you begin to play. D&S play seems to give one the munchies in between scenes, and after all the playing has stopped, everyone is ravenously hungry and thirsty. At one of my parties, a dozen people literally attacked two pans, thirty-six each, of stuffed shells, four loaves of Italian bread, and assorted sides like meatballs, cherry peppers, and salad. They licked the plates clean. And I thought I would have a few shells left over for the next day! This was after we had steadily been snacking on antipasto, Japanese hand rolls, paté, assorted cheeses and crackers, fruit, and baguettes! Then we had three different desserts, one of them birthday cake. One could hardly say I was starving my guests.

But the point is, even though, or especially because it is a party for only two, have enough to eat on hand. This would be the right time for snuggling and cuddling and sharing a bite; not the time to jump into one's clothes and run out looking for an open store.

What's in a Name?

If you don't like the name your parents bestowed upon you, this would be the perfect opportunity to be called by another name, the name of the vixen/goddess/vamp inside of you, your "mistress" name. Think of a name that makes you feel powerful and beautiful, mysterious and all-knowing. A good friend of mine, and an excellent mistress, once told me that she felt names that ended in an "a" were naturally submissive names. Why's that? Because the "a" sound at the end of a word leaves your mouth hanging open, she said. Then people can put things in it. Well, I can't tell you how I laughed at that little joke. Imagine simply saying your name and having someone stick something in your mouth! How rude! (If you're a dominant.) How sexy! (If you're a submissive.)

Pick out a name that matches the person inside of you. Then compare it to your physical appearance. Does it match? Say it out loud, and imagine yourself answering to the plaintive calls of your slave or being called by that name by others who may come to know you as Mistress. If you're five feet tall in platform heels, chances are you will not be able to convince anyone your name is "Frederique." Rosy cheeked redheads should steer clear of names like "Vertinskya." We all picture ourselves as beautiful, erotic creatures with names that announce or at least hint at our voluptuous personalities, and why shouldn't we? But our fantasy name should not be incongruous with our real appearance.

One thing I have noticed as I flip through the ads in the "mistress galleries" of different fetish papers is that the more "exalted" a title the woman has chosen for herself, the less deserving she is of that title physically. "Goddesses" weigh nine hundred pounds. "Empresses" have moles and/or warts. "Tsarinas" can crush men with their thighs. "All High Queens" are, or have, or can do all of the above. I preferred my slaves to call me "Claudia," but I would make them first say my name and then say "Mistress." I usually told them to call me whichever name sounded more pleasant to my ears. The rare ones could say both "Claudia" and "Mistress" melodiously and were allowed to answer with the one that expressed their feeling for me more accurately at the moment. If you can't think of a name that fits you, look through books. Books of names, fiction works, foreign language speaking friends are all good sources of possible ideas. Or simply have him address you as "Mistress," as I did.

The Voice of Authority

You have picked out a name that makes you feel beautiful and powerful, your confidence is up and you truly feel you can do this. What else can you do that will empower you further? Let's think about your voice. I remember reading in *Dune*, by Frank Herbert, about an order of women, the Bene Gesserit, who used their voices to control those around them. Of course this was science fiction, but whole rooms of military men stood transfixed in their places whenever one of these women used "the voice" on them. Wouldn't it be nice if you could do that, even just a little? You can. First speak in your normal tone of voice. Then drop the octave, or in other words, lower the tone you speak in. I don't mean the volume, or loudness, of your voice, what I want you to try to do is pitch your voice lower. It's not as hard as it sounds. Develop what those in the announcer business call a "confidential tone" then blend in a little firmness. Voilà, a Mistress's voice. As you and your partner become more experienced, when he hears your "mistress voice" he will know that it is time for the games to begin!

A good dominant never needs to raise her voice. Cultivate a stern look. Raise an eyebrow. Purse your lips. Look down your nose. Flare your nostrils. Tap your toe. Click your crop against your heel. Drop your voice an octave when you want to get your point across. This is my personal favorite since I have a deep voice already. Then stick with that affectation to express your displeasure, or as a warning signal that he is treading dangerously close to disobedience and subsequent punishment. The idea is to quell him with a look. My kindergarten teacher could silence the entire room by standing at the head of the class and raising one, and only one, eyebrow clear up to her hairline! Can you see how this can be fun and empowering for you?

Length of Playtime

On a more serious note, you need to decide how long your playtime will last. This will become less important as you gain more knowledge of each other's desires but in the beginning it is very important. Until you gain some experience, try not to overestimate your ability to stay in character for too long a time. There is more work to it than appears at first glance, even if you are a natural. As your slave, he doesn't have anything to do or have to do anything except what you tell him to do. You, on the other hand, have to think of absolutely everything. You have to keep him occupied the entire time you are dominating him, or make him feel as if you are. Playing the dominant can be very much like work and you are the one who has to do it.

Remember your three P's? Prior proper planning? This is where they come in, and how long playtime will last is part of the plan. You, as the dominant, should decide if an orgasm is appropriate during this session and who will get to have one. You, as the dominant, can have as many as you like. One, at the end, is enough for him. Plan on playing for an hour to an hour and a half plus extra time for that swing-from-the-chandeliers shagging you've been dreaming about for so long.

Another part of the three Ps is the method by which you will train him if he is to be your slave. You, as the mistress, are free to give him a beating because it pleases you to do so. You can also "correct" or discipline him for breaking the rules or some other infraction but something else has to be at work here. Why would he want to be good? Because he will be rewarded, of course! I favored the "reward and punishment" method myself and it is very simple. Reward for good behavior and punishment for bad. In your scene-writing efforts together, work out what will be appropriate rewards such as giving you head, the great shagging you've been waiting for, fellatio, and what will be appropriate punishments such as corporal punishment and the withholding of sexual favors.

Your Throne

I think it would help your confidence to have a position of authority from which you can survey your domain. I have used a fan-backed wicker chair, many a black leather armchair or recliner, a high straight-backed chair and the backs of slaves to name a few. Actually, the back of a slave isn't a chair, it is an ottoman, or a footstool. A chair has a back at least, if not arms; so to make a real chair out of slaves, you need two of them. A third slave would give you a chair and an ottoman, or a footstool. A fourth and fifth, an end table and candelabra, respectively.

When I was playing at home, my leather sofa (the whole thing was mine, the floor at my feet was his) had an end table (not human) next to it. On this end table, I would carefully and thoughtfully lay out each piece of equipment I thought I might like to use on him that night. I would always bring out more than I intended to use, just to keep him guessing. Of course, I made a show of it, passing each one under his downcast eyes before I laid it to rest on the table. I could feel the heat rising off him, see his chest start to heave. He would begin to pant in his desire for me. Then I would giggle. I'm a great giggler. It's so unexpectedly innocent yet what we are about to do is so deliciously wicked.

My giggle would ripple over his skin like long, sharp fingernails and goose bumps would rise on his flesh. My flesh, my flesh for fantasy.

"Now What Do I Do With Him?"

Okay. You have a lot of erotic ideas but you don't have a clue as to how to start. Start with this: exactly how will "it" start? Will you be waiting for him and call him when you are ready to see him? Will he come to you dressed? Or will he be nude and awaiting your call? If you are to make an entrance, will he be dressed or nude when you arrive? If he is dressed, how will you have him undress? Will he do a nice little striptease of his own design or will you order him out of each garment in a particular order? Will you order him in a firm yet soft voice or will you be the drill sargeant or the warden or the cop? Think about it before your first adventure because one of these openers may be the first command you give him. Be sure you have his collar or scrap of lace as his symbol of submission on hand and also whatever you have chosen for yourself as your symbol of authority.

Now that you have decided how he will arrive in your presence, why don't we continue with a walk-through playtime? And since he is undressed, may I suggest an inspection? Many men (and women, too!) find being "inspected" by the dominant to be deliciously humiliating. My favorite acceptance ritual was to have him enter my presence naked then stand three or four feet in front of me in Position Two, the inspection stance. (See chapter 11, "Positions.") Then, I would walk around him slowly, making it clear I was "assessing" him. Resuming my place on the throne, I would signal my acceptance of him by ordering him to his knees. Then, I would bring out the dog collar or ceremonial scrap of lace to bind him (or maybe even the leather wrist restraints) that had been discussed earlier.

When I used this technique to establish my authority, I made him kiss the object, be it the lace or collar or whatever else, before I put it on him. The kiss was the sign of his submission, his agreement to what we were about to do. We both found it to be very erotic. If I had a whip or crop that I planned to use on him, I would press it to his lips for the same homage before I began. If you prefer more queenly homage paid to you, Position One is not only a greeting but also a position of homage to the mistress from the slave. I highly recommend that Position One be the first thing you teach him. If you are at a loss of how to begin, it will give you something to do. Teaching him this will firmly establish your authority over him and bolster your confidence. And, if you have a penchant for ritual, as many D&Sers do, Position One will satisfy even the sternest mistress's desire for homage.

If you had fun teaching him Position One, move on to Position Two. This is the one he stood in for inspection but now is your chance to cement your control over him. Correct him as stands there, hands behind his head. Are his arms in the correct position? Is his chest puffed out, his belly tucked in? Feet eighteen inches apart, eyes down?

Since you can't have him looming over you in Position Two for the entire playtime, you might as well teach him Position Three. Position Three is a "waiting" (for a command) position and while he is waiting, you can teach him the Rules.

The Rules

Imagine that. Rules, and he must learn them. What are the Rules? Everyone is free to have different rules, suited to their special relationship, but rules 1 and 2 remain constant. My rules are quite simple:

1. I always make the rules.
2. It is my prerogative to change the rules at any time without notice to the male.
3. The male is to remain silent at all times unless spoken to.
4. The male may not look upon me or touch me without my permission.
5. The male must execute, cheerfully and to the best of his ability, all tasks assigned to him by me.
6. If the male is unable to figure out the rules, it is due to some failing or misunderstanding on his part, not mine.

Now he knows the rules and positions one, two, and three. And let's assume that you are having a great time playing her ladyship or the schoolmistress or whoever. How do you know if he is having an equally great time? Well, look at him! Does he have an erection? Is it really erect? Is there precum there? These are good things, ladies, and mean that he is most definitely turned on by D&S. Even if he doesn't need any further help in the arousal area, try talking dirty to him. Don't be embarrassed now, you're doing fine so far.

Try this in the "Mistress" voice you have cultivated: "Is that my cock, Frederick? I have a pretty cock, don't I? Nice and big and hard. And you take such good care of it for me when I'm not using it . . . but maybe I'll be using it soon." Some men prefer to be told what you are going to do to them (and you needn't be too specific your first time out): "I *do* have plans for that tongue of yours . . . but that's for later. Right now I am in the mood for some serious foot worship. I want to feel long, slow paint-brush licks over my insteps." Others respond more to the threat of punishment: "Don't expect any mercy this night, slave. We will be reviewing positions for grace and accuracy and each misstep will be severely punished." Give his manhood a soft caress as you say this (or your own version tailored to your partner's taste) and watch what happens!

Perhaps you would like to try something a little more physical, a little more hands-on than inspections, positions, and rules. Some light bondage would be fun now if he is into it. Foot worship is also good for beginners, as is dog training. Or maybe that beating from the Discipline chapter (that you have been practicing for so long) would make a good finale.

The subsequent chapters explain, and sometimes illustrate, a different fetish or D&S technique that you can explore with your partner. Cautions are included where needed, but I must remind you of this: *D&S play is rough play and the safety and well-being of your partner is of the utmost importance.* You should be expert with all the props you intend to use on him (Practice! Practice! Practice!) no matter what they are: whips, gags, ropes, blindfolds, crops, even butt plugs.

Coming Down

Remember: You have to be keeping an eye on the clock and keeping him occupied at the same time. If you are playing for ninety minutes, after seventy-five of them have passed, you will want to start to bring him down from the D&S high he is on. This is done slowly and gently—do not thrust him abruptly back into reality. A good way to do this is to tell him you are pleased with him and as a reward you will allow him to do whatever you deem or have agreed an appropriate reward to be. If his reward is to happen right then and there, after he has been rewarded remove his collar with the same ceremony you used to put it on him.

If you want, you can move from the living room, or wherever you happen to be playing, to the bedroom; if you are already in the bedroom, a move to the bed might be just the thing. How is he feeling right now? Ask him. A good D&S experience can create what D&Sers call "sub space" or put the submissive in a state called "going under." Simply put, the intense sexual experience releases chemicals in the brain that induce a "high"—a high that he needs to come down from slowly, with lots of affection from you. What he needs now is cuddling, snuggling, nesting, spooning, or some other physical closeness and sign of protection to strengthen the budding emotional bond between you. He also needs verbal support. Talk about your play. Strong emotions are at play here and if you want to continue playing, talk about what worked and what didn't and perhaps suggest scenarios for the next time.

Now what about you? How will you feel? If all went well, you will be feeling elated, powerful, beautiful, and maybe even a little vulnerable. Yes, vulnerable. This is heady stuff you are playing with here, make no mistake. This may be the first time in your life an adult ever totally and completely surrendered control of their body to you for your pleasure and you feel a little lost with this new power. If he wants to continue to play at D&S, this is the time for him to be supportive of you and to let you know that he enjoyed it. Top or bottom, people are fragile, so be careful and caring of the soul who is your partner. If he can surrender his physical body to you for D&S pleasure, his heart and mind are sure to follow. The rewards of a healthy and sharing D&S relationship are wonderful and well worth the time and effort you put into them.

You have just orchestrated your first D&S playtime and you didn't even realize you were doing it! You planned the scene, readied yourself and your equipment, established your authority and accepted his surrender, inspected him, taught him slave positions, educated him to your rules, perhaps had a more hands-on experience like bondage or discipline, then rewarded him for his good service. An entire playtime passed just like that! Maybe you could have played for another half an hour. I feel it is perfectly okay to extend your playtime for fifteen to twenty or even thirty minutes if things are going that well. As you gain more experience and communication grows between you and your partner, you can plan to play for longer periods of time. Life is short, why deprive yourself and your man of a little extra loving?

~ 3 ~

Bondage

Someone once asked me when the excitement starts for a bondage enthusiast. I replied, "As soon as they start to think about being tied up." A bondage enthusiast myself, it has been my personal experience that this is true. Bondage is so widespread that if it wasn't so nice, it could be called an epidemic. I have found bondage enthusiasts where I least expected them, in the most unlikely places, with a variety of faces from each part of the population the world has to offer.

Another thing I find interesting about bondage enthusiasts is they may have no desire to experience, or may not even express any curiosity about, any other aspects of D&S but bondage. They don't need or want to be dressed up, humiliated, or ordered around; the bondage itself is the thing. I have been with bondage fans who have gone under so deeply as to be almost unaware of my presence in the room. These people refer to their predilection as "love bondage," rather than our S&M variety.

A member of the Perverati, layered in latex, climbs into a black leather body bag and allows himself to be zipped in. Then he sits quietly, or helpfully rolls around to aid the mistress as she ties rope after rope around the body bag. A hood with tiny nose holes and little tiny goggles at the eyes covers his entire head. While the mistress sits impassively on the sofa, the man thrashes around on the carpeted floor, struggling mightily against his restraints. He heaves and thrusts his body to and fro, little grunts escaping from under his hood. The minuscule goggles have completely steamed over from his exertions, rendering him blind.

Your first bondage scenes are not going to reach this level of intensity but for many, such scenes are not unusual. The appeal of bondage lies in the isolation of the act itself. He alone is bound, with his consent, into helplessness. Consent is a very important part of this. Having given his consent is a powerful stimulant for him. After being isolated by bondage, surrendering control is easier for him because he is so obviously no longer in control. Bondage is also one of the few fetishes where a dominant will "switch" with her partner. "Switching" is when the slave becomes the master and the master, the slave.

The romance of ropes is their sensuality on the skin, the slithery feel of them, and even the little squishy-squeaky noise they make. Bondage is an exercise in helplessness; an exciting shedding of responsibility occurs once the ropes are in place. It allows the bondee to enter a separate space, isolated yet protected by the ropes. While in bondage, mind and thought processes can stop completely and one can luxuriate in the feel of the ropes on the skin. Freed from the responsibilities of the body, the mind can take new flights of fantasy.

Bondage is not only ropes; it is also handcuffs, Saran Wrap (one of those things everyone has in their kitchen) ankle shackles, velvet ribbons, stockings, leather body bags, arm restraints, waist chain and handcuff ensembles, suspension machines, fur-lined ankle cuffs, lace shoelaces, spreader bars, and a vast unnameable variety of objects that the handier bondage enthusiasts can, and often do, make themselves.

If you already own a director's chair, it's time to drag it out of the closet and buy it a nice, new black seat cover set. Perhaps even spray paint it a glossy black to give it a sleek, shiny and menacing look. It will make an admirable bondage chair and no one will be the wiser when your guests see it out in your living room. "Director's Chair Bondage" is fully explained later in this chapter.

Like most things in life, bondage can be light, medium, and heavy. To some, it can simply mean being "dressed" in ropes. To others, as tight as you can make it isn't quite tight enough. The Fetterati and Perverati know how to relax into bondage, making the feel of the ropes quite delicious and nurturing. These people sit there in bondage as happy and

quiet as clams. Others, like my latex-clad friend, love to struggle mightily against their restraints. For yet others, a Houdiniesque escape from
bondage is what thrills them. These are the ones who love to test the mistress's skill, equipment, and patience, and that the mistresses hate to see.

Mental Bondage

Bondage is an exercise in helplessness and sometimes equipment is not
necessary. Mental bondage, or "magic ropes," is an alternative to physical restraints and presents an opportunity for you to further impress
upon him his new status as your sexual slave. You can put, or order,
your partner into a certain position and command him to stay in it as
if he were tied. For those more into submission than actual bondage,
this is called "mental bondage" by some, or by the more fanciful "magic
(or invisible) ropes" by others, but it still means the same thing. Mental
bondage is different from training positions in that training positions are
assumed on command for different purposes: inspections, waiting for
commands, greeting, etc. In mental bondage, the submissive is taught to
assume a position and stay there as a humbling or learning experience.
The variation on Position Five, the kneeling inspection, is an excellent
position for mental bondage. (The position should be challenging to
hold and contain some aspect of humiliation, as in Position Five.) As he
trains himself to take and hold this position, you could give him a litany
to repeat to himself or direct him to think about past episodes as your
slave. Then, direct him to hold the position for anywhere from five minutes to an hour. Holding this position will put him in the right frame of
mind for further adventures.

Safety Factors

Bondage is lots of fun, but you should not enter it without knowing its
dangers. As the dominant partner, you are responsible for his well-being
and there are things you must watch out for and be careful of while
playing at bondage.

Even if you and your partner never progress beyond light bondage,
you must be aware of what is happening to him while you have him
tied up. A general rule of thumb when playing at bondage: *Never put a*

rope around a person's neck. Also, people with low blood pressure some-times have problems with bondage, especially if their arms are over their head, behind their back, or they are immobilized for long periods of time. To a person with low blood pressure or heart problems, twenty minutes could be a long time. Check his hands and his feet to make sure you have not cut off his circulation. If you have, they will be cold and maybe even a little blue. If this happens, release him immediately and massage the affected area until it warms up. Having him shake his hands around while they are at his sides and then over his head will help bring the circulation back. Stamping his feet will help if they are affected, too. What I do to make sure the ropes are not too tight is to slip two of my fingers between the ropes and his flesh. If my fingers fit comfortably, his circulation does not suffer. Also, if you are tying his hands over his head or tying him to something, it helps to give him something to hold on to. This could be just an extra bit of rope or a clip hook he can wrap his hands around. Suspension is exciting but has a unique set of cautions, so I would advise you to avoid it at this time.

It is important to have a pair of surgical scissors around in case your partner has to be released suddenly from his bonds and there's no time to fiddle around untying all those knots. The scissors will release him speedily and safely and give you an opportunity to discuss what the problem was. There is another thing I must caution you about while he is in bondage. *Do not, under any circumstances, put him in bondage and leave the house.* You can leave the room for a short time; many find this to be very exciting, especially when they are blindfolded as well. Later on, I describe a technique called "parking him" which you or he may enjoy. Especially you if he tends to get in your hair!

I will caution you to stay away from slipknots, especially if your slave is a struggler. A slipknot will tighten when pulled, cutting off his circulation, possibly causing him harm.

Some people fear being tied spread-eagle to anything. It is sexy to think of someone restrained in this way, all stretched out, their body vulnerable to whatever tickles the fancy and unable to do anything about it. But I have encountered many with this fear so it is always wise to ask first. Maybe having one hand or one foot free would solve the problem.

Handcuffs carry their own set of responsibilities and you should know them before you sail into the sunset in steel-shackled bliss. Keys: Do not lose them! Who hasn't heard a story about a couple playing with handcuffs, the key not to be found, the towel strategically placed, and the locksmith called? It even happened in my own building—and not to me! The doorman was playing with the sawed up remains right there at the front desk, laughing to himself about it. Imagine. But what impressed me most was that it was at only five o'clock in the afternoon.

Types of Rope

Cotton ropes and nylon ropes each have their good points and the choice is up to you. Your local hardware store will have both types so go feel them and decide for yourself. Here's the skinny on each.

Nylon ropes tend to slip. Cotton ropes don't. If your slave is a struggler, cotton ropes don't tighten up as much from slipping but do tend to make rope burns faster than nylon ropes. The most important thing is softness. Nylon is usually softer, but cotton ropes can be washed in fabric softener if they aren't as soft as you would like.

I would suggest a variety of pieces each eight to fifteen feet long. This has proven to be a manageable length for me. I don't like to look ridiculous having a length of rope so long I have to run around the perimeter of the room just to tie him to the chair. Or fussing to unravel a curly mess. You should try to appear completely in charge at all times and this doesn't cut it.

The rope, whether it is cotton or nylon, should be about as thick as your ladylike finger (three-eighths of an inch) for regular bondage. Thinner ones would be necessary for genital (cock and ball) bondage if you would like to experiment with that. You have to practice "C&B" bondage before you can do it on him. For practicing, the usual array of appropriately shaped fruit can be purchased at the vendor of your choice.

If your ropes are nylon, I suggest finishing out the ends with a hot knife blade or passing a match or lighter over them to keep them from unraveling. Make sure there are no stray fibers or sharp points when you are through. If your ropes are cotton, you may want to dip the ends in wax to prevent unraveling. If you are lucky enough to live in a maritime community, or in a city where there are good marine outfitters, check out the black nylon boat ropes they sell. Or, order them in fifty- or one-hundred-foot lengths from the Leather Harvest in Connecticut, listed in the shopping guide. These are by far the sexiest ropes I have ever seen.

Light Bondage

This is the type of bondage I would recommend for the budding dominant. Although the ties and restraints are the basic ones, they are effective, easy to learn, and easy to release, which will build your confidence for future adventures.

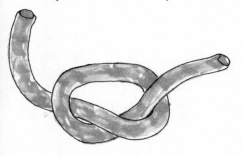

The *thumb knot* is easy to learn and useful in that it can be used to keep the rope from slipping through an eye, hole, or ring. A thumb knot is a single square knot so take the right end, drape it over the left and make a loop. Pull tightly.

ILLUS. 1 The Thumb Knot

The *Claudia restraint* is a favorite of mine (having invented and named it after myself!) that is excellent for beginners. Easy to tie, non-slipping but still allowing him some mobility to keep his circulation going, this restraint will become a favorite of yours, too. Cut a section

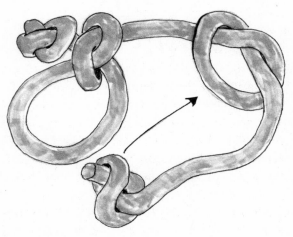

ILLUS. 2 The Claudia Restraint

just large enough to encircle each wrist as it falls at his side plus a length to pass comfortably behind his body (probably between forty and fifty inches depending on the size of your slave). Tie a hard thumb knot at each end then tie an open thumb knot enough inches up from the end of the rope to accommodate the circumference of his wrist. For instance, if his wrist is eight inches around, the open knot should be a little more than eight inches from the hard knot at the end (see Illus. 2). This knot can also be used to tie him to the bed. Attach one end to the bed frame or post and the other to his wrist or ankle.

The *square knot* is one that any scarf-wearing lady is familiar with: Fold the rope in half and place the end in your left hand over the right and tie a loop, then right over left and tie another loop. This could also be called a double thumb knot since you are performing the same action twice.

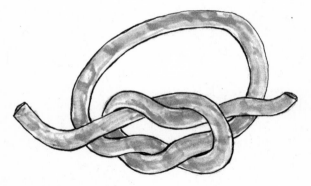

ILLUS. 3 Square Knot

And let's not forget the *bow*, a plain and simple operation exactly like the one you have been performing on your shoelaces since you were a little girl. A nice variation on the bow is *the one-loop bow*. When you make the regular bow, pull the last end all the way through and don't make the second loop. Then, you can pull the end of the looped piece to effect a speedy release. This is also called a safety knot.

Simple wrist bondage is something that every dominant should know. For this you will need a eight- to ten-foot length of rope, folded in half. Have the bondee place his palms together in front of him. The palms-together position will ensure that his circulation is not cut off because

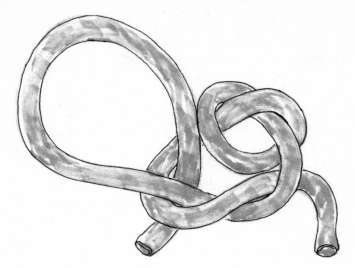

ILLUS. 4 One-Loop Bow

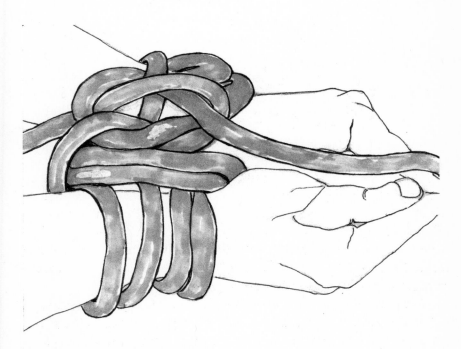

ILLUS. 5 Simple Wrist Bondage

the pulse points and veins are inside. Now wrap it around his wrists twice. Remember, don't pull it tight—you should be able to get at least one, if not two, fingers inside with his wrists. Now, cross the loose ends over each other and pass one over the top of his wrists and the other beneath them. Do this twice. Then tie the remaining loose ends into a square knot. This technique can also be used for crossed-ankle bondage.

Another nice trick with a good sturdy piece of rope is to simulate "suspension" by looping the rope around his wrists while they are in simple bondage and then tossing the rope over the top of a door. Attach the free end to the doorknob and tie. Then close the door.

To become adept at your bondage ties, use your own ankles and legs to experiment on and Practice! Practice! Practice!

Parking Him

A nice little piece of work we dominants call "parking him" is a wonderful tool to keep him out of your hair when he wants to play and you don't. He's pestering you to play, but you want to do your nails and your hair. Bring him into the bedroom, and order him to the bed or floor. Then, using the simple wrist bondage method, bind his wrists behind his back and his ankles together. Now blindfold him. Feel free to add earplugs, leave him there, and go off to do your manicure. All bound and sightless, his mind will do the work for you while you do your nails. Check on him every five to fifteen minutes, varying the amount between each check, of course, and let him know you are doing it. Say something to him or touch him to let him know you are watching over him and continue with your afternoon.

Director's Chair Bondage

Fortunately, you have an innocuous looking director's chair in the corner of the laundry room or den or maybe even stashed in the closet. Bring it out and spruce it up—ladies, this is your new bondage chair! For this piece of work, you will need two lengths of rope, each twelve to fifteen feet. Then, you can choose between the hands-behind-the-head version or the hands-bound-to-arms version.

Let's do the hands-behind-the-head version first. Sit him in the chair, feet on either side of the front legs. Have him place his palms together in front of his chest then execute the simple wrist bondage illustrated previously, up until the point where you tie it off. Now pull his hands behind his head and straighten out the remaining rope. Take one end in each hand and, enclosing the chair back in your ropes, pull them around front and crisscross them on his chest. Leave enough play for him to move his hands slightly. Now bring them around to the back of the chair. Repeat until his upper body is secured to the wooden back of the chair. You will probably only do this two to four times before the rope is used up.

On to the second piece of rope. This will secure his legs to the legs of the chair. His legs are on either side of the chair legs. Pull the rope under the seat of the chair and center it. Then loop it up through the wooden piles holding the chair arm up. Now twine it down his legs until you reach his ankles. Then put in a Claudia knot and tie his ankles and the chair leg in it.

In the hands-bound-to-arms version, he rests his arms on the arms of the chair. You begin by centering the rope behind his back, including the chair and especially the upright wooden post. Pull the rope around to his chest and crisscross in front. Then pull it around to the back and repeat one or two more times. Now take one end of the rope and snake it around and around his arm, including the chair arm in the wrapping. Tie it off at each wrist with the Claudia knot. Step two, with the second piece of rope, remains the same.

Easy Cock-and-Ball Torture (CBT)

CBT is not for everyone, so before you lasso up his willie, make sure he wants to be tamed this way. Although what I am about to describe to you doesn't hurt in the least, some men are overly protective of their parts and should be assured that the sensation is pleasurable and not really torture at all.

For CBT you will need thinner rope, rope that is quarter of an inch thick, and six to eight feet long. If he is particularly hairy, you may have to trim or shave him so his little hairs don't get caught in the rope. For all cock bondage, a hard-on is absolutely essential.

The first rope trick is one I call "All Wound Up." Totally harmless, completely unthreatening, and fun to unwrap, I would suggest you try this one on him to test the water.

Take your rope and lie it up against his shaft on the outside of his body, leaving about a six-inch piece hanging free at the bottom. When the rope is up to the bottom of the flared ridge of his head, scientifically known as the prepuce, begin to wrap it down and around his shaft. Don't pull it tight, just tight enough to stay up and in place, and make sure there are no spaces between the loops. Continue to wrap him in the rope until you reach the base

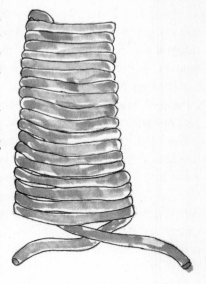

ILLUS. 6 All Wound Up

of his cock. You should still have some inches of rope left over. This you can tie to the end you left free before and hold the entire arrangement in

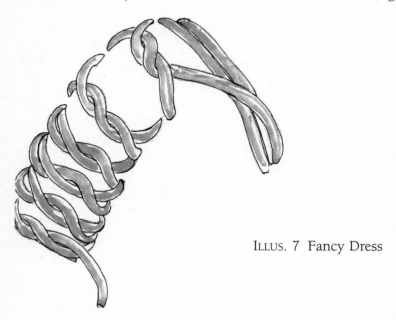

ILLUS. 7 Fancy Dress

place. When you want to unwrap him, untie the bottom and pull the long end of the rope, which is twined down his shaft. If you have done it right, his cock should do a crazy dance that amuses you and feels good to him, making his first experience with genital bondage a success.

Another rope trick you may want to experiment with is a neat little number that encompasses his sac as well as his cock. In this instance, the rope should be centered under his sac as the starting point. Then, crossing the rope ends over each other in front, the sac should be encircled at least twice with the rope, ending with the two ends back at the top. When completed, this gives his cock a look of being in "fancy dress" since it ties all the way up the front of his cock and loops off in a bow at the head.

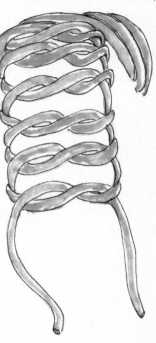

After you have looped the rope evenly under his sac twice and drawn the ends up to the base of his cock, you begin the rope trick. Tie the ropes in a thumb knot then pull them to the back. Tie another thumb knot and pull the rope ends to the front. And tie another thumb knot then pull the ends to the back. And so on and so on until you reach the prepuce, the flared ridge of his head. Then tie the excess rope off in a bow. The well-dressed cock!

ILLUS. 8 Fancy Dress

Restraints

I will use the term "restraints" to denote the myriad implements that restrict movement but do not require you to tie and untie knots.

For a partner who is tentative about ropes, check something called "Tender Tethers" or any other name implying the same thing. Essentially, they are two long ribbons with cloth cuffs on each end made of thicker, folded ribbon. The cuffs close with Velcro.

I will also explain some of my favorites that you can make from things which you can purchase in the hardware store for just a few dollars. Then

I'll move on to the wonderful things you can order from catalogues or purchase in an adult shop after you have decided bondage is for you.

Spreader Bar

One of the first things I made for myself when I was just starting out was a spreader bar. You can buy one for about $150 to $200 but you needn't make this kind of investment until both of you decide you like it. In the Preface there is a description of how to make your own spreader bar with things purchased from a hardware store. Try spray painting it glossy black to give it a professional touch. Then run the rope through the eye bolts and around his ankles. Or you can get two double-sided clip hooks and clip his ankle restraints to the eye bolts instead of tying him.

Saran Wrap

Another bondage item that tickles my fancy is Saran Wrap. Yes, Saran Wrap, just like you have in the kitchen. If you want him to stand when you wrap him, his legs will need to be about eighteen inches apart so he can keep his balance. Have him hold his hands at his sides. Starting at his shoulders, wrap the saran wrap around him a couple of times in the same place to anchor it. Then wrap it in circles around him until you reach the top of his legs. Now, you have a choice: You can wrap each leg separately or together. When you wrap him, start at his shoulders and work your way down to his feet. Then when you free him from the wrapping, cut his feet loose first so he can keep his balance. Do it slowly so you don't knock him over.

Alternatively, wrapping him to a chair or to an X-frame, if you are lucky enough to have one, eliminates a potentially dangerous fall if he does lose his balance. Wrapping him to a chair can be very sexy and the only difference is that now the chair can be included in the wrapping. Or, try wrapping him standing up with a chair behind him and then sitting him in it prewrapped.

After you have made a mummy of him, you can use your scissors to cut away the saran wrap at his nipples, exposing them for you to play with. You may also want to free his genitals in the same manner for the same reason.

Then get out the hair dryer. Using a high, hot setting, aim it at your saran-wrapped slave. Be careful not to hold it so close to him that it burns him. The idea is that turning the blower on the saran wrap will shrink it and restrict him even more. Voila! Shrink-wrapped slave. An added benefit is how warm he will get inside there, warm, wet, and slickery, adding to the sensation of being bound, not in control of himself and totally your slave.

You may want to practice this on your arm first so you will know how hot your dryer should be (pretty hot) and how close to your arm (a few inches, depending on your dryer) without melting holes in it. Or you can melt away the wrap at his nipples and free them that way. This is not recommended for his genitals, however. To release him from the wrapping, just cut him out with your scissors. Remember, when you wrap him start at the *top* and *finish* at the bottom; when you unwrap him, free his feet first so he can keep his balance.

Leather Restraints

A favorite of mine that is not in the rope category is leather restraints. This includes simple wrist and ankle cuffs, and an arm restraint that covers just his hands and wrists, or encompasses the entire arm up to the biceps. Full arm restraints feature a zipper on one side and laces on the other. The zipper side should be put towards his body, the lace-up side should face out. The laces can be used to tighten or loosen the restraint. Since his arms are pinned behind his back, his neck and shoulders or circulation may suffer. The zipper is used to free him quickly from it if this happens.

Body Bags

And my all-time personal favorite nonrope restraint is a leather body bag. This delicious piece of equipment can accommodate a six-foot-plus man on the inside and hold him safely and firmly immobilized for hours on end. You lay it out on the floor, or table, and have him climb in. Make sure he puts his arms in the inside pockets when he gets in; this will stop him from playing with himself without your permission. The body bag has two zippers, one starts at the feet and ends at the waist.

The other starts at the neck and also ends at the waist. (I imagine it was designed that way so you can torture his genitals without releasing him.) In addition to all that, there are several "D" rings up and down the outside of the bag so you can thread rope through them and pull the bag more tightly around him. As if that isn't enough, there are two Velcro flaps that expose his nipples when opened.

A new piece of bondage equipment has hit the market which is a spandex body bag. When bagged, the slave resembles a living ebony sculpture. Every curve and protrusion on his body is visible through the tight spandex. Very sexy. And, whereas a leather body bag sells for between twelve and fifteen hundred dollars, a spandex body bag costs less than two hundred. Besides, a spandex bag is washable and the leather bag is not.

Handcuffs

One of the most popular bondage items is handcuffs. They are not to be taken lightly or bought cheaply. A good pair should cost at least thirty dollars. Try to buy them at a good fetish shop. Or better yet, a police supply store. The cheap, cranky ones should be avoided. You know they are cheap just because they *are* cranky. This is not an area to skimp on if this is your pleasure.

Other than quality, another thing to keep in mind is that handcuffs are made of steel and are an "official" sort of restraint. They can cut, draw blood, and jam. You are only playing with him, not interrogating him under duress. (Maybe later on when you are both more experienced, you can play Interrogatress/Prisoner, but not yet.) So be careful not to push him over backwards onto his hands if they are behind his back or in any other position that would cause his wrists to be cut.

Some of the better quality adult stores, like The Noose in Manhattan, sell an interesting little device I have given out as a party favor many times. It is called a "universal handcuff key." It worked on the three different locks I have at home, as well as the lock on every pair of cuffs in the store. A wise investment for under ten dollars if you are not good with keys, especially little ones. In the S&M clubs in Florida, someone is always running outside to drag an officer of the law inside to free a hapless slave from a pair of suddenly keyless handcuffs! The officers, gentlemen all, are happy, amused even, to comply!

～ 4 ～

Cross-Dressing

Many a movie employs cross-dressing as a sight gag and many another puts the cross-dressed man in some predicament where he needs to be dressed as a woman for "his survival." But the usual theme in this type of movie is the "noble cause," not a genuine desire to be dressed as a woman. And the story is usually a comedy, not a drama. In the end, the hero saves the day in his girl-rags then gives them up and resumes his male persona.

If only real life were so pleasant. In my experience, and in my conversations about cross-dressing with women not into the scene but open-minded and accepting in other ways, I came to a surprising realization. The opinions on cross-dressing were almost evenly divided. One half of the women had positive reactions, the other half were pretty much against it. There didn't seem to be any middle ground for the man's benefit—just acceptance or rejection. Not one lady said it wouldn't matter to her one way or another. And the rejection was often tinged with something I can't find the exact word to describe, maybe a slight horror, or the closing of a door that a moment before was ajar.

One unfortunate man told me a story that broke my heart. He was a handsome man in a blond sort of way and dressed up beautifully as a woman. Since he seemed to know a little bit about makeup and hairstyles, I asked him if he had done this before. His reply was, "Yes, I used to play with my wife." He went on to tell me he had always had a cross-dressing fetish and one day he screwed up his courage and told his wife. To his delight, she accepted his fetish and even went so far as to shop with him for his finery. She would help him dress and apply his make-up and then they would play in the house.

"What happened?" I asked. "Why are you here if you can play with her?" He said that things went smoothly for upwards of two years when all of a sudden his wife asked him for a divorce. She confessed that at first she found it fun and kinky to have a cross-dressing husband but after some time had passed, she became unable to separate his male persona from his cross-dressing side. She felt like she was in bed with another woman and that turned her off. Turned her off to the point that she felt divorce was necessary. Her feeling was now that she knew he loved to dress, and having already done it with her many times, he would never be happy not being able to dress around her again.

Feminization, or cross-dressing, may be an essential part of a man's fantasy. Or a woman's. Then again, it might not. I don't mean to be flip by saying that; it is just that cross-dressing may never enter one's mind as part of a fantasy. You can answer for yourself. His response will be more difficult to predict unless he has given you some sign subconsciously.

Speak to him about dressing him up before you do it. If he is into cross-dressing, this may be the hardest fantasy for him to bring up on his own. You will have to go very carefully here, ladies; he may not know how to tell you he'd like to wear your panties. So try something nonthreatening and see how he reacts to it.

I once purchased for my slave a pair of ladies' silk panties and lace-top thigh-high black stockings. Although he had never expressed any interest in cross-dressing, I told him he was to wear them as a symbol of his slavery rather than his usual dog collar. I made donning the garments a ceremonious lesson, much like the ritual of placing the dog collar around his neck. Instead, the panties and hose were to signify the commencement of our games.

If cross-dressing is an essential part of *your* fantasy, but not his, you may have to romanticize it a bit for him. Many men balk at being dressed up; just as many don't. Even if all he agrees to at first is a little mascara for his long, luscious lashes (the kind few of us seem to have!), you have made progress. Tell him you always wanted to have a sister if you are an only child or only daughter. Tell him you and the little boy next door used to play "dress up" together. If he enjoys being treated like an object, tell him tonight you want to play "dolls."

If a man has a genuine cross-dressing fetish, he may not want to share it with his wife or his lover. If she knew of it before they were married, I feel their chances are better for mutual understanding. It is the rare woman who can live with a man who not only borrows her clothes but also wears them around the house.

The Total Beauty Session

I call it the total beauty session because the man who wants this type of session only desires to be dressed and made up, not in combination with any other fetish. This man is a heterosexual male, often married, who likes to dress but has no desire to physically become a woman. He will often view his cross-dressing as a "quirk" or a hobby. He enjoys it enormously except for his occasional guilt pangs about his wife.

If this is your mate's story, I hope you will consider it harmless "fun." He's not yearning to become a woman, he just wants to dress as one for a little while. Remember the questions in the quiz about playing "dress up"? If you answered "yes," then it shouldn't be too hard for you to understand.

This genre of cross-dressing is frequently combined with a desire to be treated like a girlfriend, or sister. There is no verbal humiliation, or bondage, or servitude. Often the new "girl" wants to be admired and fussed over. Popular requests are to be taught how to walk in heels, sit like a woman, cross her legs properly, and how to apply lipstick. One thing I like to do with the new woman is to teach "her" how to dance the ladies' steps in ballroom dancing. I dance the man's steps and do the "leading," sending her into turns and pulling her back, and pushing her around the room as I lead. This, of course, depends very much on her latent dancing abilities.

Interestingly, some unusual women are able to have long-term relationships with men who cross-dress. And stranger still, there are many straight, heterosexual men who are able, on a surprisingly regular basis, to meet women who can accept his fantasy and enjoy it as well.

Forced Feminization

Some slaves love forced feminization. This is when you dress him up (with his consent) "whether he wants it or not." Your reasons for this can vary. One reason might simply be that it is your desire to dress him. Or you could dress him up as punishment for some infraction of your rules. Let's say you have caught him spying on you as you disrobed. Dressing him is an ideal punishment for voyeurism. At the end of this chapter, I will give you a few tips on making up his face that I have learned from my cross-dressing friends.

Once you have determined that cross-dressing can be on your menu of dominant manifestations, you will find yourself in the lucky position of being able to dish out some mild verbal humiliation. If he likes to be dressed, tell him it's a good thing he does since he's going to be experiencing more and more of it. If he dislikes it, tell him it's too bad he doesn't like it since he's about to become more familiar with it. Tell him he's not so manly now, and his chauvinistic attitudes are about to be adjusted. (I love that part.)

Ask him how it feels to be a member of the superior sex. Tell him how lucky he is to have a taste of a woman's superiority. Prove it to him by pointing out that the advanced model, women, have interior plumbing. Get the idea? (Imagine, ladies, not only having to walk around with such a vulnerable part of your body right out there in front you but having your brains located there, too.)

As punishment, you can catch him in some act or another that displeases you, catch him being "bad." "Bad" can be anything you have agreed it to mean, from sniffing your panties to wearing them without your permission. Again, this should be discussed thoroughly beforehand.

One very popular request from the forced cross-dresser is to be turned into a sissy maid. Unlike a naked slave, this servant wears a maid's outfit and can handle a tray full of drinks at your party and then cleans up for you after your guests have left. Sounds great, doesn't it?

Forced feminization is usually accompanied by a request for verbal humiliation or corporal punishment. The perfect example would be Annabella, serving wench, chef(ess), and scullery maid all rolled into one. Annabella was all of the above at a "hen" party hosted by a friend of mine. Dressed in a sissy maid's outfit with lace frills around the hem of her dress and an apron around her waist, she was preparing a sit-down dinner for us at her own request. Her wig was carefully coiffed, her makeup neatly applied. This was an event in Annabella's life.

Needless to say, we ten dominant ladies ran Annabella a merry chase throughout the entire evening. She had to hang each lady's coat when she arrived, then bustle along to fix the new arrival a drink. Then it was back to the kitchen to prepare our dinner. Of course, she was often called away from her prep work by one of us to empty an ashtray or to fetch another cocktail. Then back to the kitchen she went to continue preparing our dinner.

In spite of all these interruptions from ten ladies, she served us an artfully arranged, and quite tasty, appetizer followed by a small salad with dressing she made herself. About twenty minutes later, visually pleasing entrées arrived in front of us, sliced lamb, potatoes, and two vegetables. Dessert was a fruit-topped cheesecake. Each course was accompanied by the appropriate wine as well as soft drinks for the nonimbibers.

After dinner, when we had "retired" to the living room to smoke cigarettes and drink cognac, Annabella was busy clearing the table and washing dishes. In between filling up our glasses and making cappuccino, that is. Then disaster struck. Annabella mistakenly grabbed the little tin of cayenne pepper instead of the cinnamon and proceeded to liberally garnish a few of the steamed milk tops with it!

Well, the ladies who got these surprise blasts were sputtering and coughing, their eyes streaming tears, for a good couple of minutes. While the rest of us were convulsed with laughter at the misfortunes of our friends, our hostess seized the opportunity to fulfill the rest of Annabella's fantasy. She invited each of us to critique Annabella's overall performance for the evening and to discipline her accordingly. Annabella was in heaven.

Each of us took a turn pointing out a mistake or infraction that we perceived Annabella had made. One lady had asked for water but did not get it. Another had asked for seconds on the dessert and didn't get it. The pepper ladies had a ready excuse to punish Annabella and did. One creative woman criticized her walk, comparing it to that of a truck driver clomping around in heels.

The punishment was any form of corporal punishment that could be performed on the buttocks. All we had in the way of equipment was our hands, a belt or two, and the shoes on our feet. I was the first one to spank Annabella with the sole of my pump. She thanked me most humbly for disciplining her and swore to do better the next time we met.

Makeup Tips

Making up his face isn't much different from making up yours. Most men, left to their own devices, usually opt for thick pancake-like foundation and pencil shadows. And forget about the mess they make with the lipstick! But we ladies know better. The main problem with making up a man as a woman is concealing his beard line and pancake make-up doesn't necessarily do this. But it always cakes and cracks and crumbles, so stay away.

First, give his face a good coat of moisturizer and wait for it to soak in completely. Find a blush that matches his complexion above his beard line. The best way to conceal his beard is to coat the skin where the beard grows with blush before you apply any foundation at all. He may need two or three coats of powdered blush before it turns the same color as the rest of his face but it will fill in. Then put the liquid foundation over it.

Of course, if he has a beard or a mustache there isn't anything you can do to conceal them. If that is the case, let's hope he wants forced feminization and not a total beauty session.

After the moisturizer and the blush coat followed by foundation, follow any course of makeup application you prefer. You may even want to thin out his eyebrows by tweezing them. Since many men do this when they get a haircut this may not be a problem but an exciting, realistic touch. A wig will add to the illusion of womanhood and should be selected with an eye toward a color and cut that will flatter the wearer. In many large wig shops a little cap can be purchased for two or three dollars which will allow the purchaser to try on the wig before buying it. If his eyes are blue, a blond or black wig may suit him as well as a red or brunette shade. Brunettes can usually wear many shades of auburn as well as other shades of brown. Wig shopping is fun and something you can do together. While you are there, get one for yourself and turn yourself into a new, different and mysterious woman tomorrow!

Gender-Swapping

Through the generations, women have been successfully "cross-dressing" as men because the public looks much more kindly on the cross-dressed woman than on her male counterpart. Sexy, and slightly intimidating in her man's suit, the cross-dressed woman turns heads wherever she goes. And with a selection ranging from men's boxy-cut suits to their boxer shorts, a woman can choose which male look, and how much of it, she wants to incorporate into her wardrobe.

I am sure many of you read the book, or saw the movie, *9½ Weeks*. In both, John buys Elizabeth an entire man's ensemble, from the skin out, including a fake mustache. After she has "dressed," she meets John in the bar of the Algonquin Hotel in Manhattan. They dine together, smoke cigars, and linger over drinks. The rest of the diners are seemingly unaware that Elizabeth is a woman and watch open-mouthed as she and John kiss and snuggle at the table. Back in the hotel room they have sex as if they were two men.

Cross-Dressing for Two

If cross-dressing is *his* thing, and you are curious about how it feels to be "the man," ask him how he feels about gender-swapping the next time you play. The cross-dressed man usually has specific ideas about his sexuality when he is dressed. He may not want you to become a man; he might want you to remain a woman so you can be "girls" together. Or he may be intrigued by the idea of being a "woman" with a "man" in a safe, planned scene. If this is the case, I have some tips to help you look the part.

The easiest part of gender-swapping is the wardrobe. Of course, many "suits" for women emulate the style of their male counterparts but for authenticity, try a genuine man's suit. Readily available in second-hand shops, an inexpensive suit can be tailored to fit your slimmer shape while hiding your feminine curves. Leave the handbag at home and take advantage of all those generous pockets, especially the inside breast pocket women's garments never have. Boots with a thick stacked-heel for the petite or lace-up flats for the statuesque complete the wardrobe.

Short hair can be parted on the "men's" side and mousse'd back or down, or combed straight back. Long hair can be pulled back in a pony-tail that sits low on the head or just atop the back of the neck. If you look good in hats, men's hats, pile your hair on top of your head, and conceal it under the hat. As you go out, don't forget to tilt your brim to a jaunty angle!

Now you have an outfit, but clothes don't make the man. When you look in the mirror, you see a woman dressed up in men's clothes. The delicate line of your jaw and your hairless skin give you away. For Elizabeth in *9½ Weeks,* facial hair added to the gender illusion. Fake beards and mustaches can be hard to handle, but beard stubble à la Don Johnson is fun and easy to apply. Only three things are needed to create beard stubble: a "beard-stubble" adhesive stick (I know the name is cumbersome but that *is* what it is called) available at costume and magic shops, a fat blush brush like professional makeup artists use, and trimmings of your hair. The hair trimmings can be collected when you get your next haircut; I asked my hairdresser to hand me the best locks instead of letting them drop to the floor. Then I put them in a plastic bag and took them home for future use as beard stubble. If the hair trimmings are too long, snip them into pieces no longer than a quarter of an inch. This length will give you a three-to-four day stubble.

The hardest part of making stubble is deciding where the hair should be. Take a look at several men's shave lines. The beard doesn't usually grow up over his cheekbones or below a certain point on his neck. Using the beard-stubble adhesive stick, draw a glue line starting at the outside of your sideburn, continue it under your cheekbone, then down toward the corner of your mouth. Continue the glue-line above the nob of your chin (and under your lower lip). At this point, you can either draw "up" the other cheek and end at the opposite sideburn, or stop here and restart at the opposite sideburn, meeting your first glue-line above your chin.

For the neck stubble, start at the inside of the sideburn, go straight down your jaw to your neck and draw the line across your "Eve's" apple. Don't worry about making this line too straight. Everyone's face is shaped differently so a little experimentation may be in order before you find the stubble line that is right to you. Now that you have your beard-stubble outline, apply the glue to the skin inside. Apply the adhesive in several coats, covering the entire area to be stubbled. If you miss a spot it will show, so be careful. The adhesive should be tacky to the touch before you apply the hair.

While the adhesive dries a little, cut the hair into short pieces. Make them different lengths, but not too long; this is supposed to be stubble. Spread the snipped hair out on the counter or piece of paper. Take the fat blush brush and swish it back and forth over the snippets. This will collect it in the brush. Starting at your sideburn, stroke the hair-filled brush down your jaw toward your chin. Repeat the process until you achieve the amount of stubble you desire.

Now look in the mirror. Adjust your attitude. Think of the way a man stands and sits and carries himself. Puff out your chest, square your shoulders. Forget the wiggle and take strides instead. Put a nice stuffed sock in your jockeys, if you think it will help. Then sit with your legs open—you have trousers on!

If he is interested in gender-swapping and is an adventurous type, why don't you suggest going out gender-swapped on Halloween? A wonderful holiday, Halloween, when everyone is allowed to wear their fantasies in the street and no one thinks anything of it. You and he can blend into the crowd of revelers, no one the wiser for the secret you share.

~ 5 ~

Discipline

I think people pair bondage with discipline because the words sound so nice together. Bondage and Discipline. It does have a ring to it. But a discipline enthusiast can have one without the other and not feel in the least deprived. They are two entirely different things: Bondage is mainly an exercise in helplessness whereas discipline is being corrected or punished for some infraction, like breaking a rule. There are so many types of discipline, so many reasons discipline is desirable, and so many ways to discipline him that everyone will agree discipline merits a chapter all to itself.

"But I love him, I don't want to hurt him," you protest. First, stop whining. This is fun! Since we have already established that D&S is *never* done in anger, and you are not mad at him, you can take out all of the latent hostilities built up by your day on his pink little hide. Secondly, you can beat him without really hurting him or leaving any marks.

Corporal punishment seeks to achieve many things. One is behavior modification and it explains itself. Conditioning can be an aspect of corporal punishment. You can train your slave to associate pain with a certain pleasure by giving him both at once. If you stroke his genitals while you pinch his nipples, he will still get an erection. He will come to associate the gentle caress of his privates with the pinch and soon you won't need to stroke him. The pinch will achieve the same effect. Another thing corporal punishment seeks to achieve is sensation; in this case, pain. Pain is neither good nor bad, it is just another sensation. Some are excited by it, others are not and then, there are some who are excited by it but may be unwilling to admit it.

Discipline is an intriguing subject. For many of the "old school," discipline is a clear sign they are worthy of correction and discipline, and that discipline made them better people for having had it. In older generations, a spanking, paddling, or caning meant the receiver was loved and cared about enough to be disciplined. These early childhood associations die hard, if at all.

At one time, I was seeing so many white-haired, blue-eyed, bushy-browed elderly English gentlemen who wanted canings that I bought a few extra in case one broke in mid-session. (Then I found a canemaker whose canes didn't break: George Hinson-Ryder from Santa Fe, New Mexico. See the Shopping Guide.) Often these canings were combined with other aspects of D&S. In one instance, the gentleman wanted an elaborate scenario told to him about the new regimen of corporal punishment I was going to inflict on him to make him a more worthy slave. A major ingredient of the tale was how many times a day he would be caned and when, and in what position. Then some verbal humiliation was thrown in for good measure.

The most common form of discipline is corporal punishment. It can take the form of a spanking, whipping, caning, paddling, or cropping. In this chapter, I will discuss the different types of corporal punishment as well as touch on noncorporal punishment. I'll give you the general themes, an anatomy lesson, and describe, step-by-step, how to conduct a beating properly. But the most important advice I can give you is Practice! Practice! Practice!

The Anatomy Lesson

Before we go any further, we are going to have an anatomy lesson followed by a lesson on how to practice with certain instruments. The anatomy lesson is important for everyone who hopes or intends to conduct a beating during playtime. By now you know that you can hurt your slave unwittingly if D&S play is not practiced with knowledge and common sense. Common sense you already have; the anatomy knowledge will be given here. You need to know about his body because that is what you will be playing with. Take care of it!

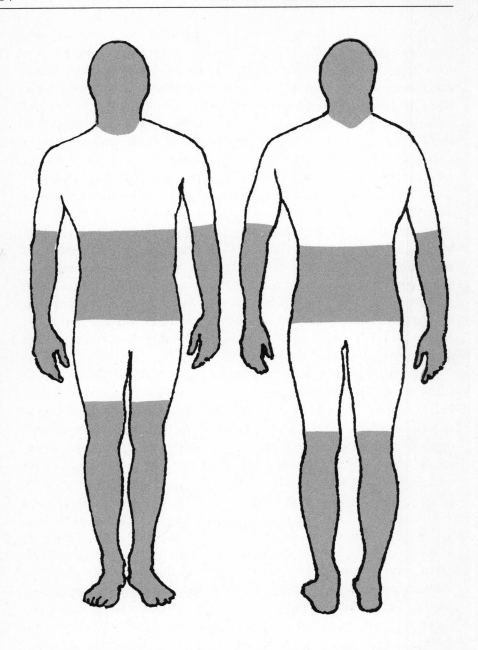

ILLUS. 9 Safe Areas and No-Go Areas for Discipline

Look at the line drawings of the human body. They are the front and rear views, and we will use these drawings to demonstrate which areas are safe for beating and with what. In both the frontal and rear views, the dark areas are off-limits for anything but gentle stroking. The light, or unshaded areas, are generally safe for a dominant with sense and anatomy knowledge. *A general rule of safety is* never *to hit the eyes, ears, nose, or mouth, or any bone joints, ligaments or internal organs. Never hit above the neck with anything other than your hand.* Look at his body and assess it for what it is: some have more fat than others, some more muscle, but everyone carries their padding in a different place. The padded areas, which we will get to in detail, are usually safest.

To the frontal view from the top, the first dark area, his head. Consider the head the domain of the Perverati as there are many cautions to delivering a slap in the face. The jaw can be pushed out of joint from an improperly delivered slap. Aim for the most padded part of the cheek instead. Since neck problems can result from the head snapping around (like a form of whiplash), you should hold his head with your other hand to prevent injury. Make sure he wants this before you reach out and assert yourself.

A surprising number of men find it highly erotic to be slapped in the face by a woman. Upon request, I have delivered a number of well-placed slaps to the most padded part of the cheek, of course. Several years ago when Ava Taurel and I taped a segment of the Maury Povich Show, a man in the audience, a very brave man since this was national TV, stood up and said it was his fantasy to be slapped in the face by a woman. Ava was off the podium in a flash. Bounding up the stairs to where he stood at his seat, she grabbed him by the front of the shirt and Pow! Pow! Let fly. Forehand and backhand, one for each side of his face. The audience was shocked into silence. He thanked her very sincerely and sat down dazed, noticeably retreating into a happy place inside himself during the rest of the show.

Let's return to the front view of the body, the unshaded chest area. If your partner has good pecs, is a body builder, or is just well cushioned there, he may enjoy being whipped lightly on his chest. Aim for his breasts and have him tilt his chin back to avoid stray lashes catching him in the face as they land. Remember that chests cannot be hit with the force that the buttocks can. And, if the top of his chest is bony, he may not enjoy being whipped there at all. Just use your fingertips to tweak and pinch his nipples.

Now we move down to a shaded NO GO area. This is the middle of his torso, his belly and abdomen, and his genitals. I would avoid the middle of the torso completely as there are many vital organs underneath. For the Perverati, the genitals might be a different story. Many submissives find a gentle genital whipping with a soft, short whip to be highly pleasurable. But this is not for everyone. As sensations in the genitals can vary greatly in just a small area, changing from pleasurable to excruciating in a millimeter, extreme caution should be exercised. Start gently with your lightest flogger and if he likes it, build him up to a harder one later. But genital whipping is considered to be an art in itself and best left to the Perverati.

The next light area is his thighs. Although unshaded, these areas require expert aim since there are many major tendons between the legs and the pelvic area. These are close to the surface in his groin and should not be hit. Besides, it hurts like hell and a lot of people don't find the sensation erotic. The hip area should also be avoided as there is nothing erotic about a beating there.

The last part of the front view is from the knee down. This part of the body is all bone therefore off-limits to any hitting or instrument.

Now for the back side of the body, and the good news: this is where most hitting, heavy or not, can be done. And the bad news: there are still things you must be aware of when hitting the back. Let's dispense with those at the top first. *Never hit the back of his head, his neck, or spine.* A heavy blow may fracture some vertebrae but the common danger is from inflammation triggered by repeated hits with even a light whip.

The first good area is his upper back and shoulders. Some submissives express a preference for this area. The upper back is very muscular, very strong in a man and hence, a wonderful place for whipping. The muscles there are often tense, especially if he works out or uses a mouse, and a good whipping can be like a D&S massage. In this area, only a "whipping" in the literal sense, with a whip, will do. Some like a caning or a cropping here but not many. Most prefer only the whip on their upper backs. And since this a large target, it will be easier for you to land your strokes in the general area. The only caution is to avoid the spine and the protrusions of his shoulder blades.

The dark area below his shoulders, his middle back, should be avoided totally. This is where his kidneys and other soft organs are located. Boxing fans will tell you that kidney punches are illegal and with good reason. We don't want him urinating blood next morning, do we? Avoid the area from the bottom of his ribs to the top of the crack of his ass (the ilium, or pelvis).

Now we can move to the best part: his delectable, hittable buttocks and his upper thighs. The butt is one of the most pleasure-laden areas and since padding here is almost guaranteed, its the safest place to beat, and beat hard, on his whole body. So let's talk about the butt first. So round and cute, getting all warm and red, squirming and wiggling, so near the asshole and genitals, butts have inspired countless millions of kinky people over the millennium. Sade-ists, or Sadians, as in afficiona-dos of the Marquis de Sade, are great butt lovers, idolizing the rear and rear view over the front on both men and women. Like the upper back, butts can hold lots of tension. Butts are great for spanking, whipping, caning, cropping, and paddling. A good beating relaxes the butt, as well as the anal sphincter. This will be important if you decide to experiment with anal play.

Even with the butt, you should exercise your good sense and look at the butt being offered up to you. No two are alike. If he is thin and bony, he must be treated differently than someone with a large, well-padded rear end. The part of his butt, be it thin or well-padded, just below his waist and above his crack and around the sides towards his hips should be avoided.

Each butt has a "sweet spot," a spot where the muscles are thick and deep and can take a good beating. Get him on all fours then think of his ass as a target. Although the exact location of the sweet spot varies from person to person, it is usually found on either side of the crack, low on the butt, in the area right around the anus. Put a bull's-eye there, with his anus as roughly the center of the target. The bull's-eye ends right below his coccyx (tailbone). As you move farther up the bull's-eye towards the coccyx, the blows become less pleasurable but they still feel good. Approaching the tailbone and above, the muscles and fat thin out and it is very painful when this area is hit. You wouldn't want to break his ass, would you?

Let's move on to the backs of the thighs, the next best area. Although thighs are usually padded and therefore safe, thigh hits hurt more than ass hits. My favorite place is neither ass nor thigh, but what I call the "fillet" and others the "sweet meat." It is the crease where the butt meets the thigh and an interesting spot, indeed. Since this lovely little bit of flesh moves each time he does, a bruise there would be hard to ignore, wouldn't it? Think of him sitting there in his car or on the train, this little bit of flesh rubbing against his trousers which in turn are rubbing against the seat. And then what would he be thinking of, my dear? You!

As on his front side, the area from the knees down is pretty much off-limits. As are the arms and hands. The only exception could be the bottom of the feet. This is the domain of the Perverati but it is also an official form of torture called the bastinado. I doubt your first-timer is asking you to take it that far. A soft whipping with a short, light flogger can be very erotic but it must be soft. There are many delicate bones in the feet and the tendons are close to the surface. The feet take the weight of the body every day. Think of how good a foot massage feels and if you can make your whipping feel like that, give it a try.

There are some cautions. For your purposes, the main two concern paddling and caning. During a paddling or a caning, your slave is usually bent over something, an ottoman, the arm of a chair, even your lap, when punishment is given. These positions are preferred since they offer up his butt and present a clear target for you. However, in these positions, his tailbone is right below his taut skin, not in its protected cover of cheeks as it is when he is standing. If you just nip the tip of his tailbone, you could certainly put him in distress for a few minutes. If you hit it hard, he could be sore and uncomfortable for months. Worst case scenario, you could bruise or chip the bone. You've heard the expression, "she broke my butt"? Well, in this case it would literally be true.

Spanking, Whipping, and Caning

There are many general things about the discipline that I would like to address before getting to the particulars of spanking, whipping, and caning. You have already found some things in your home that can be used as instruments of discipline. When you went on your treasure hunt you probably found a hairbrush, ruler or yardstick, wooden spoon, spatula, the sole of a pretty slipper, a sports paddle, and his belt. More, if you are imaginative or have a very well-stocked home. Perhaps you have a bona fide instrument of torture from an earlier fantasy and foray into D&S. However, if the belt strikes you as the most realistic instrument of torture, be sure to practice with it on a pole or the coverlet first. Belts are much harder and trickier to use than you think. A small investment of under twenty-five dollars will get you a crop from the local riding outfitters or a cane from the local fetish store. Regardless of the instrument, there are certain procedures, or steps, to a good beating.

Sensitizing the Area: No matter what instrument is used for the beating, sensitizing the area you are going to devote your attention to is highly recommended. Not only does this prepare him for the beating he is about to receive, it also establishes a rapport between the two of you. Properly preparing him for the beating will assure him of your skill and your awareness of his well-being.

Sensitizing can be done in any number of ways and can be matched to the instrument of discipline if it pleases you. A spanking is an intimate beating, with him across your lap perhaps, so I would suggest you smooth your cool or hot palms across his cheeks, or trail your fingertips or dragon lady nails lightly over his butt, hopefully raising goose bumps. Then use the palm of your hand to smooth the goose bumps away. Do it more than once, more firmly each time.

For a whipping, try using the tresses of your long hair, brushing it over his back and buttocks to erotically sensitize him. A long millinery feather is one of my favorite things too. Since you are using a whip, use the ends to sensitize him. Hold the whip perpendicular to his butt and dance and trail the ends back and forth across his prone, and loving it, body.

If you are using a crop, especially a braided leather one, it will have an almost snakelike, scaly feel when slithered back and forth across his exposed flesh. Or, try playing it like a cellist's or violinist's bow across his hard member.

Now that he is ready, willing and eager for this beating, what are you going to hit him with? Let's talk about multilashed floggers, the easiest to use and purchase and many a top and bottom's instrument of choice.

Instruments of Torture: The best gentle whips, or "lightweight floggers," are made of soft hides such as deerskin, elk, and light cowhide. Deerskin is the preferred choice here as it is velvety soft, makes a big, loud noise, and packs little to no wallop. Therefore, it is a perfect "warm-up" whip since it raises the temperature of the skin but doesn't hurt him. A deerskin whip is like being caressed by so many soft fingers. These whips are perfect for people who are not into pain but more into the sense of being dominated. Elk and cowhide are a little heavier than deerskin and can be used the same way as a deerskin flogger. A horsehair whip, which doesn't hurt but has more of an abrasive effect, can be used as a warm-up whip as well.

If you get lucky and he turns out to be a full-fledged masochist, by all means go for the "heavyweight flogger"! Although it is called heavyweight, I would classify this type of flogger as moderate on the pain scale. I say this because I am not physically strong enough to swing this flogger hard enough to make it anything more intense than moderate. But used with a light touch, this flogger can do double duty as a warm-up whip as well. Floggers in this category can be made of bullhide, bison, or moose.

In general, any whip made of stiff lashes should be avoided. So should latex or rubber whips. Single-lash whips are for the Perverati and one of them will be happy to instruct you in its proper use. (Try practicing it on a tree in your yard!) *Always* test the whip on yourself before you use it on someone else. The budding domina may want to consider ordering a matched set of floggers from Janette Heartwood at Whips of Passion in California. She can help you if you are unsure about what works best for you, and her catalogue is a delight. Janette's whips feel good in your hand: the balance is there, the lashes are soft and plentiful. They are well worth the investment.

On to canes and crops. There are no such things as "gentle" ones. These two can be wielded gently but will always leave some sort of mark no matter how lightly you apply them. Both come in varying lengths and thickness with the cane being harder to use and control than the crop. The cane requires lots of practice and unless you are willing to put in the time, leave caning in the realm of the Perverati. A crop, however, is much easier to use than a cane and that cute little "keeper" or flapper on the end is fun to play with, without actually hitting him with the rod of the item.

There are many other exotic instruments of pain that fall into these general categories that are interesting to mention although you may never see or use one. The most popular would be the single lash whip. But there are also signal whips, bullwhips, dog whips, quirts, bamboo rods, bastinados, and on and on. Most of these are very hard to use and are very dangerous unless used properly. You must have someone in the Perverati teach you the art of these objects because you can even hurt yourself with them! And then Practice! Practice! Practice! My suggestion: stay away until you have much more experience and an experienced teacher.

Cautions

Marks: Some love a souvenir; others are appalled at the faintest hint of red. Some implements, like a deerskin flogger, leave very faint marks that are gone in an hour; others, like the cane, leave welts that last for as long as ten days. Marks can be lessened by getting him into a queen-size pair of pantyhose (best for a flogging) or by placing a damp washcloth over his butt (better for a caning).

Testing the PQ (Pain Quotient): The best way to test the pain quotient of a whip is to try it (gently!) on yourself. No one can adequately express to you how it feels and one stroke is worth a thousand words. We haven't discussed the savage variety of whips here, only the gentler types you are most likely to use. To test a cane or crop, try it on the palm of your hand. This isn't the best test, but it is almost impossible to cane yourself effectively.

Wrapping: The ends of the flogger have a tendency to curl around his body and hurt him in the most unpleasant way. This wrapping, as it's called, occurs when you overshoot the mark. The tip of the whip is what hurts the most and leaves the worst marks, so you must learn to control where it lands. To avoid wrapping, a simple measurement of your arm plus the flogger, much like the measurement used for caning, is advised.

In the beginning if you constantly wrap him, try putting a pillow next to his far side (this only works when he is lying down) to absorb the tips. Better yet, take a step away from him. Practice! Practice! Practice! If you are constantly wrapping him, you are standing too close to him.

Practice Techniques

Spanking/Paddling: A spanking or paddling requires very little training. Your hand, with or without the paddle, will tend to go where your eye sends it, unlike an instrument which can be affected by the flick of a wrist or a twisted lash. So if you intend on spanking him, you needn't worry too much about your aim. A good spanking requires only a practiced hand. And a good spanking will sound like one. The blows should not sound monotonous and should be rhythmic in their own right.

The paddle, however, is much more brutal. Butts are the only place that can stand a paddling so limit its use to his ass. If he is bent at the waist for the paddling, and his scrotal sac is in danger, invite him to protect his jewels by covering them with his hands. Avoid the tailbone area and aim for the fillet, or underside of his ass, for safety. The category of "paddle" includes not only the classic schoolmistress's and frat house wooden paddles but also a variety of leather goods such as slappers, smackers, strops, and straps.

Caning/Cropping: To practice with a cane or a crop, use a pillow or a cushion that has some sort of pattern on it. Squares or stripes are terrific for practicing because you can clearly see where the blow has landed. Stand up straight but relaxed and to one side of your target. To measure the length of your arm with the cane or crop in it, hold the instrument comfortably in your outstretched hand, elbow flexed. Place the instrument where you want it to land and adjust your position by moving your feet away from the target. The tip should overhang his butt by only one inch to avoid "wrapping."

Then, take aim, a deep breath, and strike. Note where the tip landed and where the cane or crop creased the pillow. Now, try to place another "mark" a quarter of an inch below your first one. Try again and again, and not only today but other days, until your blows are consistently landing where you aim them.

Whipping: To practice with a whip, you need to know some "whip strokes" to practice first. I have included several in the following pages. The stance is the same as caning/cropping except that now you will be facing your target, either from the side or directly in front of (or behind) him. Some of you will automatically know how to handle the whip when you get it in your hand and for you, I have included more advanced techniques. The punishment positions are covered in the "Positions" chapter.

The *overhand* is an all-purpose stroke that goes from warm-up to heavy in intensity, and is very easy to learn. Take the whip in your hand and let your hand fall naturally to your side. An overhand stroke relies on the pivoting of the arm at the shoulder, so, as you swing your arm up and around to the back and then over, your palm will naturally face down when you land your stroke. I don't want to overexplain this action because it is more natural than you think and with practice you will get better.

The *forehand/backhand* stroke is easy to learn and provides a moderately abrasive feel. This is a good stroke for when he is bent over something, his butt offered up for a target. Since this is a back and forth motion, only the tips of the whip will touch him, hence the abrasive action. The horsehair whip made by Janette Heartwood, is excellent for this. Grasp the whip easily in your hand, extend your arm, and forehand and backhand him across the butt in much the same motion as a slap in the face.

The *circle* is an easy-to-learn warmup stroke. Done from the wrist, the idea is to pinwheel the ends of the whip at his butt. This is usually used as a warm-up stroke because it is difficult to put great force behind a wrist stroke with a flogger.

The *backhand/overhead* stroke is another "all-purpose" stroke, which can range from gentle to severe, and requires some degree of skill. Starting with your hand held naturally at your side, whip and palm in, bring the whip across the front of your body and up over your head. As the whip passes over your head, catch the lashes in your free hand to right them and immediately let them go so the whip can make its arc and land the palm-down, backhand blow.

The *figure eight* stroke ranging from warmup to abrasive, requires supple wrists. This is like the forehand/backhand stroke, only now you are making a figure eight with your wrist. This blow is more for abrasion than pain since no great force is behind it with a flogger, and it can take some time to perfect. It is very showy but has little effect, as it tends to land on the side of the buttocks rather than on the meat.

The Elements of a Good Beating

Now you are conversant in some types of whips and several whipping styles, as well as the human anatomy. The practicing is done and we can move on to juicier things. As you have guessed by now, there is a lot more to a beating than just waling away at his bottom. Most beatings start with a sensitizing of the area. You have wafted your feather, fur mitt, or bunny cloth over his buttocks, tickling him a little as you do so. Then you progress to lightly dragging your nails over his flesh. Now dance the ends of the whip over him. If you are using a cane, soft warmup strokes, spaced at least five seconds apart, will sensitize him. If you are spanking him, use your bare hand. Sensitize the whole area you will be punishing. Doing this will let him know this area is about to receive your undivided attention. Use the above techniques or invent your own.

Whatever you are hitting him with, begin by hitting him gently and use the first stroke to test your aim. If you are too close to him, step back. If you are using an instrument and not your hand, find out what "gently" is by testing it on yourself. Start by hitting him gently, just warming him up a little, making playful little slaps or strokes. Alternate between the caress of your fingertips and the blow. This is still the beginning, you have to work up to the harder blows by increasing his tolerance level slowly. After a few minutes of this, eliminate the caress for five to ten light strokes, then caress him once more. Repeat at this intensity, caress him, then make the next ten strokes a little harder. Caress him again. You can increase the intensity of the blows in stages of ten or twenty between caresses. These techniques can be used to begin a beating with a flogger but not a cane, crop, or paddle.

Note: If you are spanking him, ten strokes may be surprisingly hard on your hand. You may want to reduce it to five spanks at a time.

The only real limit to how long the beating lasts is the stamina of each of you. For your part, giving a beating is work—make no mistake! If you start out slowly and use the sensitizing techniques, build up to it properly and sustain the sexual tension, a good beating can last for two or more hours.

This would also include little breaks for you to see to your own comfort during that time. You may need a drink of water especially if you are talking to him while you beat him. If you have ice in your glass, take out a cube and drip it on him or run it over his hot butt cheeks. Or, you may need to use the throne room. Also, you will need to change strokes to prevent an affliction D&Sers call "whip shoulder," which is similar to tennis elbow and computer neck.

In regards to your slave, the beginning of the beating will be very nice for him. All that feathering and finger-trailing and tickling. Even the first twenty or thirty strokes will feel good to him because they are just light ones. The next twenty or thirty strokes should be a little harder with an underlying bite to them. As the beating gets harder, he should be trying to keep still under the blows but *not* be in real agony. Remember, if it hurts, you're not doing it right.

Many factors can affect the quality of a beating. One of the main factors is the position he is in during it. If he is facedown on the bed, his buttocks and his whole body are relaxed and the beating hurts less. This is the most comfortable position for the slave and I recommend it for the budding domina. On the other hand, if he is bent over the arm of the sofa and his cheeks are stretched, the beating hurts more.

The place where the blow lands also plays an important role in the quality of the beating. There is the high, round part of the cheek and then there is underside of it where the "fillet" is located. Hitting the high round part where a lot of adipose tissue is located stings more; hitting the fillet or the underside of his cheek engages the muscle rather than the fat. When you hit the fillet with a nice underhand stroke, like you are bowling a strike, his whole butt quivers in a cheek-quake that is absolutely adorable. This is more noticeable during a spanking or paddling.

The Elements of a Good Spanking

For spanking fans, it will be more interesting for both of you if you not only move the blows around to cover the whole cheek but to learn different types of blows and their effect. Try starting with short, light slaps that progress to short stinging ones. Then try a "landed" blow, a blow where the hand lands and stays rather than snaps back up for the next one. Experiment with light, medium, and heavy landed blows. Next, try "flipping" the four closed fingers of your hand at the fillet. You can also vary the rhythm as you hit him: one left, one right, two and two, then three and three. Spank each cheek separately then spank both together from the underside and quake those cheeks!

Your slave will find it more exciting if you talk to him about what you are doing. The official D&S term for talking dirty is "verbalization." Many people are turned on by dirty talk and since he can't see it for himself, make a visual for him. You can start out by describing how white and pale his cheeks are and how red they are soon to be. Then, as you spank him and they begin to get a faint pink glow, talk about the pink glow. Use the word "pink" a lot, pink being on the road to red. When they become red, describe the red to him too.

You can also use the comparisons of cool, warm, and hot cheeks as the beating progresses, either alone or in conjunction with the white/pink/red spiel. Try this: How cool and white your cheeks are now (trail your fingers over them) but soon . . . then begin the beating. As his cheeks turn pink and warm up, talk about their warm pinkness. If he likes his beating to progress to hotness, an ice cube tip trailed across his flaming buttocks will cool him down and give him a nice surprise.

A spanking may be his choice of corporal punishment simply because he perceives that while he is lying naked over your lap he will have the opportunity to rub his genitals on your thighs. This should not be allowed. Any action like this requires your permission first. If the purpose of the spanking is punishment, he should not be getting pleasure by rubbing on you. He should be made to hold his hips up off your lap by making an inverted V of himself. If he repeatedly fails to hold this position, use it as a lesson in position training at a later date. In the meantime, place a cushion between you or make him assume a position over the arm of a chair or end of the sofa.

I like spankings on the one hand and on the other, I don't care for them too much. I like them because they lend a personal touch and a really good spanking definitely softens up your slave. I don't like them because they are extremely hard on my hand. While spanking my slave on one occasion, I broke a nail and bruised my middle finger so badly that it swelled up like a balloon and sported a big, ugly, black and blue mark for a week. The effect on his ass, however, was negligible. I also find that my hand hurts from spanking his bottom long before his bottom hurts. My hand also hurts long after the spanking has worn off. This is hardly the desired effect.

The Elements of a Good Caning

A caning or cropping is right up my alley. He gets to be in an uncomfortable standing-up position, my hand and manicure are preserved, and the cane makes more of an impression (both physically and psychologically!). A mainstay of masochists and the Perverati, the cane takes some degree of expertise to use. Caning is very severe, always leaves heavy marks, and is not for the average beginner. Most newcomers do not want this high degree of pain. To use a cane properly and without damage to your slave, you must Practice! Practice! Practice! (As described on page 72.)

So now your aim is true. Before you land your first stroke, flail the cane through the air to find its "sweet spot." Each cane has one and to find it, just keep turning the grip in your hand and whoosh the cane through the air. When it makes the proper whooshing sound, you will know it. That is your cane's sweet spot. Your aim will be better when you find it and direct it "facedown" at his buttocks. Additionally, the whooshing sound a cane makes is unmistakable and your slave will come to love and hate it. It will send shivers up and down his spine as it cuts through the air.

Now use the cane itself to warm him up. Tap his butt lightly with it. These are light, flicking taps you're giving him here. Play the cane across his cheeks as if they were the strings of a cello or violin. When he is nicely pink and warm, flick at his butt a little harder. These will be the middle strokes. Keep looking at his bottom, no matter what you are beating him with. It will tell the "tail" of what is happening to it even if he can't. How does it look? Like it's had enough? If it does, stop. If he asks for more, continue if you think it is advisable but proceed with caution. He may not know how much he has taken or can take. He is new at this too.

Deep into the domain of the Perverati now, we progress to administering the hard strokes. The hard strokes should be placed one above the other starting right below the fillet and ending (as he is bent over) on the upper curve of his cheek. Leave several seconds between each stroke. If you read him well and can see when his buttocks have relaxed from absorbing the previous blow, you can strike him again then. Cane him slowly! Canes strike deep and welt on two levels. There is the initial pain when the cane lands and welts the upper skin, then a few seconds later a new deeper pain flares out from the cane stroke on the muscle below. This pain flares up one's spine, electrifying it, then explodes in the brain like a white hot twin sun going nova. Too many strokes delivered in rapid succession spoils the beauty of the double pain and defeats its purpose. Because of the exquisite nature of the pain a caning gives, many masochists favor this type of discipline.

The maximum number of hard cane strokes I would recommend for the beginner is six. You can slowly increase it to eight, then ten, then twelve. I like to pause before the final two strokes and ask him if he is "ready" to receive them, or if he "wants" them. Then I give him my two best shots to remember me by.

If you are beating him for fun, there is nothing wrong and everything right with stopping to kiss him or caress him or rub your mons Venus against his charmingly presented bottom. I beat Slave Frederick for fun regularly, often to hot music so that our "affectionate" time often resembles dancing. If he is bent over something while you are beating him, grab a handful of his hair (hold it close to the scalp and get a good handful, not a few strands) and pull his head back. This will arch his back and press his hot bottom into you. Dance and move around, holding his head by the hair, in between your lashing groups. Slave Frederick and others love the highly sensual combination of a beating and lap dancing for the mistress.

Noncorporal Punishment

Noncorporal punishment is obviously more subtle and requires a deeper understanding of your partner for it to be effective. What is punishment for one barely affects another. Punishment of this type is closely tied to humiliation. For the man whose mother used to dress him up as a girl when he cried, forced feminization is punishment. To another, being made to perform an act he hates, like cleaning the bathroom, is punishment. If you have assigned him some task to perform as a punishment, stand over him and supervise. And, in your best dominant tones, don't be shy in pointing out what he is doing wrong and correcting him. This doesn't mean screaming or cursing, use your dominant tone of voice and perhaps express some disappointment over his failures. Maybe he will feel guilty enough to perform better the next time.

Inventing things as noncorporal punishment is like going on a treasure hunt in his and your minds. You will find elements of noncorporal punishment in cross-dressing, foot worship, little-boy fantasies, and many others. Being made to sit in a corner in a dunce cap, wear a diaper, write one thousand times "I must not displease my mistress," being given dinner in a dog's bowl, being made to sleep in a cage or on the floor—all this is noncorporal punishment. (The very interesting subject of humiliation and head games is discussed in chapter 9.) While anal play can be very sensual, inserting something into his anus can be a punishment and a very humiliating one, at that.

~ 6 ~

Exhibitionism and Voyeurism

Exhibitionism

When I say "exhibitionist," I don't mean the classic flasher in a raincoat with the cutoff legs of trousers taped up above his knees, exposing himself to unsuspecting passersby. An exhibitionist in the D&S context could be a dominant who enjoys demonstrating the obedience and training of her slave in a public setting, or a submissive who enjoys being used in this way. A submissive exhibitionist may also enjoy being forced to appear scantily dressed, or be disrobed or displayed in the nude, then commanded to perform any number of services or entertainments for the mistress. Many people who are basically shy in their regular lives use exhibitionism in the D&S context to free themselves from societal or emotional dictums that stifle their fantasy life and sexuality.

There is a contingency of male dominants within the D&S community who maintain that any woman who is an exhibitionist is a submissive. They love to make these sweeping statements that have no basis in fact other than that is how they would like it to be. Anyone, male or female, can be an exhibitionist. Some are exhibitionists who know absolutely nothing, and couldn't care less, about D&S. In the D&S setting, the mistress leading her submissive into the club or play area on the leash, clearing space to play and then setting up and enacting her scene, is an exhibitionist, not a submissive. When I pointed this rather obvious fact out to the macho men, they stared at me blankly. It seems they overlooked this point.

For the submissive, being exhibited by the top can fulfill any number of fantasies. The submissive can feel exhilarated and deliciously embarrassed by being made to appear scantily dressed in public or to walk nude around the house. Commanding him to assume a bent or spread position and expose himself to the gaze of the mistress can have him panting in mere seconds. A large number of men that I have spoken to have described fantasies where the mistress keeps the slave naked, forces him to assume positions that expose him to her view and others, and uses his body as a toy. This could be for further training or the mistress's enjoyment, or to impress upon the submissive the mistress's control over him either in private or in public. More importantly, the fantasy will emphasize the elements of control and power exchange that its creators enjoy the most.

In the submissive male sense, when I say "play in public," I don't mean only taking your mate out in full drag in broad daylight. There are many more subtle ways to exert your control over him in an exhibitionistic way. You could have him wear your panties under his suit when he goes to work or when both of you go to dinner. Call him at the office and inquire about his undergarments. While in a cab or car, have him show them to you.

No one knows exactly how many exhibitionists and voyeurs there are in the world—no one polls these things except in research studies too small to be applied accurately on a global level. I would think that with rare exceptions, people in the performing arts have a bit of the exhibitionist in them. Stage fright or not, once under the lights and in front of an audience, soon all jitters evaporate in the warm glow of appreciation and admiration from the onlookers.

Being an exhibitionist led to my first appearance as a panelist, along with two of my friends, on CNBC's "Real Personal," hosted by Bob Berkowitz. The segment was simply titled "Exhibitionists." It has been suggested that, since the show was broadcast live, I had more guts than brains but I think the exhibitionist in me won out. There I was on live television, a station with fifty million viewers, chattering away about how I liked to flash shoe salesmen. And how I had sex with my lover at a party while the guests watched. And how I'd like to walk out onto Second Avenue in New York City and hail a cab wearing nothing but a mink coat and high-heeled pumps. The show garnered very high ratings and it was often shown in reruns. Of all the shows I have appeared on, "Exhibitionists" is my favorite.

I think I became an exhibitionist when I got my kindergarten diploma and walked across a stage for the first time. All the smiling, upturned faces, the lights, the applause—I was hooked at the tender age of five! After that it was on to dancing school for ballet and tap and, oh heaven, the recital at the end of the year. It was then I noticed that the adults in my child's world recognized my comfort in the spotlight and deliberately put me in it. When there was a school play, I always had a good part, if not the lead. If announcements needed to be made, the mass narrated, speeches given, I, with my deep voice, was always picked to stand at the front of the auditorium and speak into the microphone.

I think that if you are an exhibitionist and an exotic dancer, you have found your calling in life. It is the perfect job for an exhibitionist. I do not agree with the fire-breathing feminists who say that exotic dancing exploits women. That is only one way of looking at it. I feel that the dancers are exploiting the weaknesses of men and enjoying every minute of it. There you are, showing off your beautiful body and strangers are giving you money for the pleasure of looking at it.

Perhaps exhibitionists are born, not made. But I definitely do not agree with those who say exhibitionists are latently submissive. Is the dominant woman submissive when she gives her slave a beating in an S&M club? Hardly. She is secure in her ability to dominate him for the enjoyment and titillation of the onlookers. She is proud of the way she looks in her dominant gear. And she wants to be admired for her skill and expertise. Her slave feels pride in her for exhibiting not only her control over him but also in her own individual style as a dominatrix.

A good example of a relationship between two exhibitionists is the one I had with Sam. The theme for the first play party I ever threw was the "Half-Naked Party." Not only did I think being half naked would encourage people to mingle and play together but also because my apartment is unbelievably hot, and fifteen people would not be comfortable in there unless they were only half dressed.

Realizing that you have to give your guests something to do other than just eat and drink, especially if you do not have a real dungeon to play in, I decided to give the ladies a whipping lesson, using the perfect party toy, Sam, as a demonstration model. I put Sam in bondage with my then-boyfriend Mickey's assistance. I enacted the sensitizing and the full range of blows, explaining what I was doing as I went along, just as I explained it to you earlier.

Then I invited each lady to take up an implement and try her hand on Sam. All the ladies stood to the side as the first domina made her initial swing, corrected her aim, and made the next. Every lady got her chance. By the time the fifth lady was up at bat, the blows were definitely less timid. The sixth lady had Sam pulling on his restraints. The last lady, who had some experience with D&S, made him say his safe word.

Sam loved being the demonstration model, loved beatings, and loved all the attention he received by being the perfect party toy. For myself, I love sharing something wonderful with my friends, love being in the role of teacher/mentor, and love all the attention I receive while doing both. A match made in heaven.

When Brianna, my straight drag queen friend, and I used to make forays down to the old Vault, in Manhattan, we would find ourselves a sofa in a dark corner and make out. Crowds of men would gather around to watch us kiss while they touched themselves. We were exhibitionists since we knew a mistress kissing a drag queen would draw a crowd. Those who gathered to watch were voyeurs.

On another occasion in the Vault, I met a very handsome young man named Simon. Simon was a real newcomer, who had come to see the players play. He was so green, he couldn't tell the real women from the drag queens. I caught his eye and signaled him to join me. As soon as he sat down, the first thing he said was, "Are you a real woman? Some of them look so good, I couldn't tell they were men." (I said he was green.) I assured him I was the genuine article and began talking.

As fate would have it, we spoke during the week and made plans to see each other over the next weekend. We wanted to go back to the Vault. He was fascinated by what he had seen there and wanted to experience more of it and perhaps even participate or put on a scene. I was delighted.

When we arrived, we found a sofa on a high platform in the back playroom that was empty. We arranged ourselves so we took up the whole thing and no one could climb up there and join us. (I like to be looked at and admired, not touched.) Then we began to kiss. I have a passion for kissing when it is done well and Simon did it very well. Both of us were getting very hot from kissing and when he lifted me into his lap, I helped him get me there.

This was a great scene. I was wearing a black halter dress with a full skirt and thigh-high stockings and a garter belt and high-heeled black pumps. Simon tossed my full skirt aside so my black stocking thighs and the creamy white skin above my hose were visible to the onlookers. He stroked the outside of my leg down to my foot, then back up to my thigh again on the inside of my leg. His other arm held me firmly against his chest and his lips moved from my mouth to my neck.

My arms were flung around his neck, and my head was thrown back as his breath and lips kissed my throat. I arched my back and bent my leg at the knee as I clutched his hair, pushing his face and lips into the curve of my breasts. Simon pulled aside my panties and began to trail his fingers ever so lightly over my wet pussy. Then he plunged his tongue into my mouth at the same time he plunged his fingers into me. The voyeurs couldn't actually see him doing this but they knew what was going on. They gasped in collective lust, envious of the passion they were witnessing.

Simon and I were very hot at this point but we never lost sight of the fact we were putting on a show. We were aware of it every second we were doing it and did it up for the viewing pleasure of the onlookers. Like true exhibitionists who knew they had put on a good show, when we were through, we simply rearranged ourselves and got up and left, excited and high from our little show.

Voyeurism

Voyeurism is the flip side of exhibitionism. Many people are voyeurs and don't even know it. If you live in a large city where walking is a common means of transportation, chances are you are a voyeur in a mild sense of the word. Do you look in people's ground floor windows as you walk by? When you are sunbathing up on your roof, do you look around to see who is on the other roofs? Or, if you happen to glance out your window and see a neighbor doing something interesting or unusual in their apartment, do you discreetly watch for a few minutes? Or are you and your man really into it, and have binoculars and/or a telescope? Would you have enjoyed watching the scene in The Vault? Even one yes answer qualifies you as a voyeur.

I have spoken with many men who are voyeurs in the D&S context of the word. This type of fantasy embraces some sort of spying on the mistress, combined with a specific punishment when caught in the act. The spying could occur when the mistress is in her bath. Or it may occur as she is getting dressed, or putting on her makeup, or when she is relieving herself of her golden stream. In short, he likes to spy on you when he knows you are performing a private act, an act you wouldn't let him witness under normal circumstances.

The punishment for voyeurism varies with the individual. The most popular are forced feminization, corporal punishment and humiliation, or a combination of the above. If forced feminization is the punishment of choice, bondage may also be introduced since you are forcing him to dress. And then a little verbal humiliation comes into play. You could tell him about his punishment as you inflict it upon him.

Let's say you have caught him "spying" on you while you dressed. He is peeking through the crack of the bedroom door, panting with desire. You hear him, run to the door, fling it open, and surprise him. Feigning anger, grab him by the arm and pull him into the bedroom. This will be easy to do even if he is much bigger than you since he will be cooperating. The more earnest mates will assist you in the physical acts to compensate for their larger size. However, if he turns out to be a ham, overreacting to everything, discipline him immediately.

So now you have pulled him into the bedroom. You should be saying things like, [indignantly] "Spying on me? [slightly menacing] Do you know what happens to [adjective of choice, nosy, dirty old, unworthy] men who spy on me? [then, with a she-devil, icy smile] I'll be delighted to tell you." Then do exactly that. Of course, this has been discussed in advance and you have agreed upon the punishment.

If forced feminization is to be the punishment for spying, as we spoke about in chapter 4, "Cross-Dressing," then he may want to be made more into the caricature of a woman than a passable one. Humiliation plays a large role in this fantasy. (Don't get caught spying on a girl, or else she'll turn you into one.) Don't be too careful when you apply his lipstick. Dress him up in clothes that look really funny on him, lots of lace or frilly, very feminine things. Put pin curls in his hair and hold them in with bobby pins. Then make him look into the mirror, hold him by the arm (perhaps you have thought of putting one of your more feminine robes on him) and tell him how stupid, or ridiculous, or foolish, or ugly, he looks. He will have to tell you his preference so you don't say the wrong trigger word. Or laugh at him, if he is overly sensitive to it.

～ 7 ～

Fetish Wear

No matter if you rank among the Glitterati, the Fetterati, or the Perverati, one thing they all have in common is the love of fetish wear. Millions wear clothes of a fetishistic bend and have absolutely no interest in D&S. Even Seventh Avenue fashion designers have "done" fetish wear, and who knows what *those* people are into!

Fetish wear is an important facet of the D&S scene. Most of the better S&M clubs enforce a strict dress code at the door and go so far as to tell you what you can wear in case you can't figure it out for yourself. Certain members of the Perverati are exempt from the dress code for reasons of skill, longevity in the scene, being a legend in their own time, or just because they are a special friend of the manager.

All joking aside, D&Sers spend a great deal of time and money on their wardrobe, saving up and/or shopping for months to get just the right outfit for the ball with the perfect accessories. That goes for the men as well as the women. In D&S-land, fanciful dress is de rigueur and men are as likely to pull out all stops as their female counterparts. Bored with their everyday wardrobe of suits and ties, the D&S man can tailor a fashion statement to please himself. Leather pants, ruffled shirts, and silver-topped walking sticks for the "lords," latex or full leather outfits and whips for the "masters," frilly maid's outfits complete with apron and cap for those who love to serve, and police or military uniforms for those who love to be in control.

For women, the selection is even more spectacular. The white-robed princess and the black-clad evil queen; the slinky, sexy femme fatale and the metal-clad cyberdomina; the strict schoolmarm and the corsetted, petticoated saloon girl all live happily side by side in Fetishland. Lingerie one night and leather chaps the next, fetish wear and playing "dress up" is an important part of D&S. We women are lucky that footwear plays a large role in the mistress's wardrobe. What more of an excuse is needed to go shopping for shoes? But male or female, fetish dressers are a flamboyant lot and their manner of dress helps them to establish their group identity.

The Leather Mistress

I know men who love to see a woman dressed in leather but have no interest in D&S. Millions of people who wear leather aren't leather fetishists. But then again, maybe they are and just don't hang that label on it. What is the fascination with leather? Is part of the lure of leather that it suggests a philistine paganism, a wanton dark side, a mysterious aspect to one's personality?

Leather is like no other material in the world. It has its own aroma, nothing else smells like it, or feels like it when you have it on. Kind of tight and stretchy at the same time. Some wear it because it's glamorous. Others because it's "tough." Some may wear it for protection, like a biker guy. He may not have a fetish for it but he certainly develops a fond appreciation of it after wearing it through a fall or during cold weather.

I love leather. I have been wearing leather (and getting odd looks from some and longing and admiring looks from others) for twenty-five years, long before it was mainstream fashionable. My own current leather wardrobe consists of a full-length ball gown, a minidress, two pairs of pants, two skirts, two vests, a motorcycle jacket, a pea coat, a blazer, and about half a dozen teddies. Bras, G-strings, garter belts, opera-length and over-the-elbow gloves, three pairs of boots of different heights (below the knee, just over the knee, and thigh high), and a cap complete the head-to-toe-in-leather look. Oh yes, I just purchased a nice leather sofa, chair, spanking bench, and ottoman. In black, of course.

Leather wear is not only popular with mistresses but also as apparel for slaves. Their wardrobe is much skimpier than yours—they are slaves and as such, they are not entitled to wear anything at all unless you give your permission. Leather wardrobe for male slaves includes G-strings or thongs, body harnesses (full or half), vests, shorts, and chaps. Of course, any of these can be worn by the domina as well. But remember, as the dominant partner, you get to wear more than he does. His nakedness is a symbol of his servitude.

A Leather Session

Your slave is in his place, on his knees at your feet. Try beginning with a command to sniff the hem of your pants. Talk to him about the leather, its smell, its texture. Now direct him to massage your calf through the leather of the pants. Have him move up and rub his nose on your leather clad thigh. This can be done sternly or playfully, depending on the tone you have set ahead of time.

Many leather fetishists love to be commanded to perform cunnilingus on the mistress *through* her leather pants. I have no words to describe how this feels. He has to work very hard at this because the leather is thick. And it is usually very tightly stretched across your crotch and your pussy is right up against the leather on the inside. But from your point of view, the harder he has to work, the better it feels. It's as if the leather intensifies the sensation because of its thickness rather than inhibits it. Exhort him to lick it hard, baby, and move that tongue around!

Latex Lovers

Latex and its lovers seem to be more popular in Europe than they are here so American latex fans tend to attract a lot more attention than their leather counterparts. I'm not saying that is why I like latex but I'm not excluding it either. For those who are unsure about what latex is, I call your attention to Michelle Pfeiffer's catsuit in *Batman Returns*. That's latex. And Ms. Pfeiffer looked wonderful in her suit. It's more expensive than leather and harder to take care of, needing special washing, powdering, and storage.

Wearing latex is like being naked when it's cold or in a sauna when it's hot. Since you have to get all powdered up to get into the garment, and you have to powder the inside of the garment itself to get it on, all that sweat and powder combine to make a paste on your skin that has to be showered off. Additionally, it has a peculiar odor, as does the latex polish. So why, you ask, does anyone bother with it?

Nothing feels like latex, not even my beloved leather. Or my darling shoes. Latex is sort of "upper crust" because it's expensive. I think it denotes a certain amount of seriousness about D&S. And it makes me feel so sexy. It clings lovingly to every curve (rendering an aspirin visible in your stomach!). It makes a squeegeelike noise when you move. You see nothing yet you see everything. It makes you highly visible and gives you an aloof mystique. It is an attention-grabber. Strangers walk up to you and inquire about your garment. It's great.

Late one Saturday night, I squiggled into a latex dress, shined myself up, and went out to get a cab down to The Vault in Manhattan. A cab was coming down the opposite side of the street. I didn't think he saw me standing there, all dressed in black on a dark night. But the cabbie saw me, all right. A native of Germany, he espied the shine of my latex from up the block and across the street and cut across three lanes of traffic to pick me up before anyone else did. He initiated conversation—the topic was my dress. The entire ride was spent discussing latex, its look and feel, proper care, and where to get it. When we arrived at The Vault, I got the feeling he would have rather accompanied me inside than go about his business.

Although latex is very expensive, a miniskirt only costs about seventy-five dollars. A black top of any sort will do to start. An added benefit, if you are concerned about wearing hides, is that latex is a one-hundred percent man-made material and no animal has suffered or died to make it.

Rubberists

A breed apart from latex lovers, rubberists carry their love of wearing latex to an erotic extreme. The client I described in "Bondage" in the multilayer latex garments and bodybag is a rubberist. A man I buy fetish clothes from is a rubberist. Often spending thousands of dollars on wardrobe and rubber sheets, the rubberist completely encompasses himself—head, feet, hands—in several layers of latex then sits around and watches television. Or maybe goes out. To the rubberist, the wearing of the latex is the thing, not the staying in or going out in it.

The safest sex imaginable can be had by two, or more, people in latex. A rubberist friend told me that his idea of really good sex is two people in latex catsuits rubbing (no pun there) on each other until both achieve orgasm. For some reason, the mental image of this strikes me as very funny.

Caring for Latex

The most dangerous time for your latex garment is when you put it on. It is very important that you take the time to powder yourself and the garment so you can wiggle into it with the least amount of stretching possible. Gather the latex in your hand the way you would a stocking and role it up your body. Watch out that your fingernails do not rip it or poke a hole in it. If possible, turn the garment inside out and roll it up your body. Then peel it off the same way.

Latex has to be properly cared for in order not to ruin it. You will have to hand wash it with a mild, *nonoily* soap in a tub of warm water. A good swishing will remove the powder. Rinse it in cool water then dry it completely inside and out. You can hang it over the shower pole stuffed with towels or you can dry it manually. When it is completely dry, powder the inside lightly.

The following are things that are no-no's for latex. Heat of any kind. Do not use hot water to wash it, do not use a dryer or any other heat generating object to dry it. Strong detergents will affect the bonding in the seams and they may eventually let go. Prolonged exposure to light will fade most colors. Oils from your hands will discolor white and pastel latex so try not to touch the garment too touch, or wear gloves. White and pastel latex should not be stored with black or dark colors and contact with metal or jewelry can spot the garment. Products with oil in them will severely damage latex. (In this regard, treat it like a large condom. They are made of the same things.) *Do not* use furniture polish on your latex. Use only products that are made for latex.

Hanging is not recommended for latex since it stretches. Keep this in mind when you buy it. Many stores hang their latex. Latex garments that are hung will eventually have problems where the garment meets the hanger. I place mine flat on tissue paper (acid-free is best, if you can get it) then put a second layer of tissue over the garment. Folding it carefully, I make sure no part of the latex touches another. If it does, more tissue. Not doing this will cause the latex to stick to itself and when you try to unfold it, you will rip it. Then store it in a cool, dark place.

A Latex Session

Latex, because of the care involved, presents a large variety of tasks that you can assign to your slave. First, he can assist you in the powdering of the garment, and/or of you. Then he can help you into it. After it is on, you will notice that a lot of the powder that was on you is now on the dress. Give him a washcloth wet with *warm* water, instruct him to wash the powder off the garment, with you in it. Next, you have to be dried—give him a soft, lint-free towel and set him to work. Notice how these actions feel like a massage—nice perk, don't you agree?

Now that you are depowdered, washed, and dried, you can present him with the latex shiner and a soft cloth. I recommend "Black Beauty Latex Polish," available in a pump spray for convenience. Usually, some sort of cleaning and/or shining product can be purchased at the same place where you buy latex. A word of caution: I have wooden floors and have found that errant sprays of latex polish on a wooden floor are very slippery. As in fall-down slippery. So if you have carpeting or a rug, I would suggest standing on it while he sprays the polish on.

Then tell him to polish you up. Keep up a verbal diatribe as he does it: You want to be so shiny, you can see your face reflected in your latex-covered lap; you want to squeak when you walk; you missed a spot; what about my seams, don't they deserve to be shiny, too?

After you sit, the shine will have come off, leaving you with a big dull spot on your derriere. If you are going out dressed in latex with him, give him a little bag containing the polishing cloth and polishing liquid. His duty will be to reshine your dull spots during the evening, making sure you are looking your best all night. And finally, the washing, drying, and packing for storage "ritual" can become his responsibility.

~ 8 ~

Foot Fetishes

Feet are feet and some people will never understand the fascination. And after looking at some men's feet, it is not hard to understand, well, their lack of understanding. Most men really don't take any time or trouble with their feet, hence some look like poached flounders and others like horny toads. It is an unusual man who sports a nice, sexy foot at the end of his leg, and when he does, it turns me on. Women fare better in the beautiful foot game. Even if the woman's foot itself is not beautiful, things can be done to bring out its beauty, or at least make it more appealing. Frequent pedicures can make a big difference not only in the physical condition of the foot but in your mental outlook regarding your feet. It's hard to feel that your pampered feet, with their soft, fragrant skin and freshly painted toes, are anything but pretty when they look so well cared for.

Foot worship usually includes a fancy for toes, soles, arches, insteps, dainty ankles, shapely calves, silky, or silk-stockinged, thighs. Or they might like combat boots, shiny vinyl boots, boots with heels, boots with laces, suede boots, or boots with ridged soles. I remember when "your mother wears combat boots" was an insult. Now it's a fashion statement. Or the preference could be for any type of shoe imaginable from penny loafers to sneakers to pumps to fetish stilettos. Perhaps the interest lies in the foot itself: a long, narrow aristocratic foot, a big, wide foot, and a very petite foot. Or maybe a foot whose second toe is longer than the first. At least you won't get bored because there are an infinite number of varieties on the foot theme.

At first I was puzzled by the origin of this fantasy. One can assume that the older English gentleman who likes caning likes it because he was caned at school. Or a little boy is dressed as a girl because he cries like one. But feet?

So I asked three people I knew well in the mistress/slave sense what started them on the road to foot worship. Their answers were all variations on a theme. Each of them, as an infant or child, had been placed on the floor to play at Mommy's feet. All they saw of Mommy was Mommy's feet, calves, and shoes. It was as if a cartoon light bulb appeared over my head. Of course! There were some differences in that one mother wore nude stockings rather than black. Another's mother wore a girdle and high black stockings. The third's mother wore black patent leather, pointy-toed pumps. His mother used to "play" with him using her foot. Teasing him into trying to catch it, she would get it away just in time, letting him catch it only once in a while.

Indubitably, there are many men whose fetish did not start this way. Maybe they started out as a "leg man" and came to appreciate a pretty, well-shaped, soft foot at the end of it. Or any one of a whole large city full of variations. Although the variations are endless, what you need to get started is relatively little, and some of it you already have.

F'Etiquette

A well-cared-for foot is of the utmost importance. Your nails should be smoothly clipped or filed to the length most flattering to your toes. Your polish should be fresh, not chipped. If you are prone to callouses, especially on the balls of your feet or heels, a pumice stone on a regular basis will alleviate this problem. The pumice stone works best when both your foot and the stone are wet. Some salons use a moisturizer on the pumice stone. Then, use a lotion to moisturize your feet just as you would any other part of your body.

Since your feet are attached to your legs and most foot worshipers also have an eye for legs, a freshly shaved or waxed leg is a must. Stubble is not desirable unless specifically requested.

Next you need shoes, preferably black, in leather, patent, or suede, in that order. If you do not wear hides, a pair of peau de soie pumps will do very nicely for you, if not him. The shoes should look expensive, and not be run down or in need of lifts, soles, or a shine. As high a heel as you can manage and still be elegant and commanding without twisting your ankles is advised. Plain pumps, pumps with ankle straps or ankle laces, open-toed pumps, sling-back pumps, spike heels, mules, high-heeled sandals, boots to the knee or higher with a heel will all accomplish the same effect. Now, you *do* have one of those things in your closet, don't you? I thought so.

Now you need hosiery. Black is always popular, followed by nude. The sheerest, silkiest ones you can find. Stockings and a garter belt are recommended unless you know for a fact your man likes pantyhose. And garter belts drive men wild. If you are like me, kind of slender, the garter belt may slip down over your hips. This makes, as we all know, "elephant knees" in your hose. A big no-no. So I buy lace-topped thigh-high stockings and wear them with a garter belt. They stay up because of the grippers, not the garter belt. The belt ends up being more like decoration, but he'll never know!

Then there are those whose passion is pantyhose, or fishnets, or even slouch socks. If he is a pantyhose fan, my only caution to you is: Make sure the seam in the panty is arranged flatteringly. In other words, line it up directly with the crack in your cheeks to present a sleek, well-dressed appearance.

Let's continue getting dressed for a foot session. Your legs and feet are ready, now we need the rest of your outfit. Remember that you are the mistress. Although he will be seduced by you eventually, he is there to submit to your will, to be your slave. Lingerie is popular as wardrobe for domination but I don't feel it is necessary for a foot worship session. So wear an entire outfit; you are under no obligation to show him your body even if he is your lover. Then you can tease him half to death when you show him an extra inch of thigh.

Any type, style, or cut of bra you feel most powerful in is what you should wear. If you are not as busty as you would like to be, pick up a padded bra or some Cadillac pads (available from the Frederick's of Hollywood catalogue) and make some cleavage if that will empower you more. There is also a very sexy selection of bodysuits available in lingerie shops and through catalogues. Thong or full-backed, many are made in sheer black nylon or lace and look absolutely mouthwatering with thigh-high, lace-topped stockings.

Now for your bottom half. I would suggest a miniskirt in any material, cutoff dungaree shorts (another favorite with men), a high slit skirt, tights, or anything else that shows off your legs in all their glory. This selection is entirely up to you.

I often opt for a third piece to cover the bra or top. If I am not wearing a dress, only a skirt and bra, I usually wear a lace jacket or leather bolero over it. Then I take the jacket off partway through the session. As in any session, he is not allowed to look at me unless I give him permission.

Foot Worship

Now you are dressed and have discussed the scenario beforehand. The music is on, the candles are lit, the answering machine on, the cat out, whatever. You need a signal to establish when the games have begun. As I suggested earlier, a dog collar ceremoniously placed around his neck is a good signal. Or you could ask him in your "mistress voice" if he is ready. Use the same phrase all the time until you both get the feel of things. Then he should be able to tell by the change in your attitude, or your tone of voice, that you are ready to begin.

Another approach is to order him to undress, either privately or in front of you, whichever you prefer. If he is a good dancer, have him do a little strip for you. Tell him what you want him to take off first, then next. Aesthetically, I prefer shirt then shoes and socks, followed by his pants, then undershirt, and finally, his underpants. Tell him that in the future you don't want to see his clothes in a disorderly pile; he's to fold them neatly and put them out of sight. Then have him assume the position of servitude at your feet that you have worked out earlier.

I have very hard wooden floors so I have a round chair cushion that I refer to as his "lilypad." When he is not doing something on my command, that is his post and I expect him to be on it.

Instruct him to get down on his knees and then have him sit on his heels as in Position Two. Be sure to point out to him that his knees should always be open, making his genitalia available to you at all times. His hands should be clasped behind the small of his back or resting palms down on his thighs in Position Three. Next, you can inform him that you want him to address you as "Mistress Claudia," or whatever your preference is. In the chapter "Slaves and Slave Training," I will give you helpful hints on how to have a well-trained slave.

Now you should be ready to give him his first command. If you are without a clue, tell him you want a foot massage. I find this to be a very good way of determining my slave's sensitivity as well as a good way to stall for time while I think of what I would like to have him do next.

If his technique is unsatisfactory, correct him. When he does something wrong, let him know. Explain to him how you want it done. Demonstrate on his hand and then have him do it to you. Allow him to kiss your arch if he shows improvement. Give him ten lashes if he doesn't. Then reiterate your instructions and have him try again.

If his massage technique is good without much coaching from you, he may have a natural aptitude for massage. Lucky you! You can train him to give you pedicures (saving you a small fortune at the nail salon) and your toes will always look delectable to him.

Massages can be given to either bare or stockinged feet, depending on the preferences of you and your slave. Some will only deal with the stockinged foot. Others prefer only the bare foot. The smart ones love both. I say this because there are so many more things you can do with feet if the bare is also included. Especially if he likes a little humiliation to go with his worship.

The Foot Bath

One of my favorite things to do with the bare foot is to order my slave to give me a footbath. This is a wonderfully relaxing treat for you, and special for him too, if he is a foot fetishist. You'll need one of those cute little foot whirlpool things. I have one—a gift from an ardent admirer. My favorite scenario goes something like this.

I sit in my throne in the living room with a latex sheet under my feet (regular terry cloth towels will do). My slave has laid out the scented soap, the pumice stone, moisturizer, and the towel to dry me. Then he comes in with the footbath already filled with soapy water and kneels in front of me with it. Before he is allowed to place my feet in the water, he must test it to make sure it is not too hot. Since he is a foot fetishist, he has an enormous hard-on because of the proximity of my feet. I order him to test the water temperature with his erection. If it is too hot, he will remember the next time. Then I order him to gently place each foot in the warm, soapy water. I direct him to lather up my toes with the scented soap, paying special attention to the succulent crevices between each one. He moves along the sole of my foot, massaging me with the soap. Cupping my heels in the palm of his hand, he massages me in a lovely circular motion I taught him myself. He uses his thumbs to massage the skin around my ankle.

I have trained him so that his touch is relaxing and soothing, never tickling. When he is through washing me, he uses the pumice stone on my one lonely callous, taking care not to remove it completely. Then he gently removes each of my feet from the footbath and pats it dry. Now I am ready for the warm lotion. I have him heat it in the microwave for a minute before he is allowed to use it on me. No cold moisturizer on my feet! Of course, he is still throbbingly erect and tiny beads of pre-come glisten at the tip. Why not put this to good use? Have him add his warm goo to the heated lotion and massage both of them into your feet. It is a nice treat for him if he has given you good toe service.

My favorite way of rewarding him is to press the soles of my feet together creating a hollow that his "lotion holder" can slip in and out of. Then I talk to him. I tell him I expect a sizable deposit because he has been storing up for so long; that I expect many pumps, all perfected targeted, and not a drop wasted on the sheet. I tell him that I am impressed with the quantity of lotion and allow him to massage the lotion and his warm goo into my foot.

"Catspaw"

I have another little game I like to play and if you are a cat person, I'm sure you'll enjoy it, too. It's called "Catspaw." I get to be myself or the Mistress or whoever and he gets to be the cat. He is curled up at my feet purring and rubbing his head on my ankle. I reach down and scratch him behind the ears and talk to him in "cat talk." I call him "pretty kitty" and "little bag of bones" and ask him if he would like a treat. My kitty follows me into the kitchen rubbing against my legs as I walk. I return to the living room with a quart of warm milk and a large shallow bowl. I place my feet in the bowl and pour the milk over them. Cats love milk and mine is no exception. My kitty licks all the milk up; up from the tender creases between my toes, all around my foot, all of it, until it is gone. And if he has been a very good kitty and not left one drop of milk in the bowl, I bring him up onto the sofa with me. I lick the milk off his whiskers and scratch his favorite places. Then I allow him to use his sandpaper tongue to give me a lovely orgasm.

Toe Games

Another favorite with the bare foot is to pretend that your toes are like fingers. Playfully grab his nose between your big toe and your second toe the same way you would if you were using your index and middle fingers. Then gently shake his head back and forth, propelling the motion with your foot, the same way you would using your hand. This is the "isn't he a (good, cute, obedient) little slave" line of reward. You can use your toes to manipulate his lips, open his mouth, turn his head. Sit on the far ends of the sofa facing each other then you stretch out. Place one foot on either side of his nose, covering his eyes, cheeks and mouth with your foot. Teach him to suckle your toes, one at a time. A gentle nibbling on the ball of the foot can be deliciously erotic. Another nibble on the pad under the big toe will send shivers of delight up your spine. Slipping a finger in-between each toe and spreading them is a welcome release after pointy toed shoes. As you become more comfortable with your play, together you will think of more things to do that you both enjoy.

When you gain some experience, I would highly recommend walking on your slave. Some D&Sers call this practicing trampling. This is a sure thing for the ardent foot fetishist. I mean it *never* fails to excite him! For this, you will need some way to support yourself as you climb on him and stand. Once you are actually standing on him, your balance will not be very good since you are walking on a squishy surface. I have a chin-up bar installed in a doorway where there is enough room for him to lie underneath me. No one ever guesses what I really use it for unless they are foot worshipers themselves. A lot of people ask me how many chin-ups I can do and I just smile enigmatically and don't say any-thing. A mirror is also installed on the opposite wall so he can watch the action when I am not standing on his head.

The Anatomy Lesson

Next we will have a short anatomy lesson because if done incorrectly, you could really hurt him (as in breaking a rib) if you mount and walk on him incorrectly. This anatomy lesson is different from the one in "Discipline," so please do not skip over it.

Look at the line drawing of the human body titled "Safe Areas and No-Go Areas for Standing." It is divided into six parts. The first part is his forehead. Part two begins at his eyebrows and ends at the bottom of his neck. Area three starts at the top of his chest and ends below the nipples. The fourth part is his rib cage and stomach. The fifth is from his hips to his genitals. Area six is his legs and feet. His arms and legs are unsuited for slave-walking although an occasional finger-trodding will remind him who is in charge.

Areas Two, Four, and Six are the primary danger zones. Regarding Area One: *Never step on his cheeks or jaw.* They will not support your weight. Additionally the lower jaw bone, the mandible, is movable and stepping on it could dislocate it. Regarding Area Four: *Never step on his rib cage and avoid his solar plexus.* The ribs are somewhat flexible and protect his diaphragm and his lungs. Your weight on them could cause the ribs to snap. Worse case scenario, they could snap and puncture a lung. As I said earlier, his arms, legs, hands, and feet are unsuitable for walking.

Area four also contains his stomach. Although I am unaware of any particular safety risk in a normal healthy male associated with walking on this area, some men simply do not like the way stomach-stepping feels. Perhaps the sensation is painful, or their stomach muscles are not up to the pressure, or maybe they have just eaten. But I have found this to be something that the slave either loves or hates so if he is uncertain, try it once and be guided by his reaction to it.

On to the good parts: Areas One (his forehead), Three (his chest bone and nipples), and Five (his hips and genitals) are the leading sec-tions for body walking. In Area One, the skull is a hard bone and can

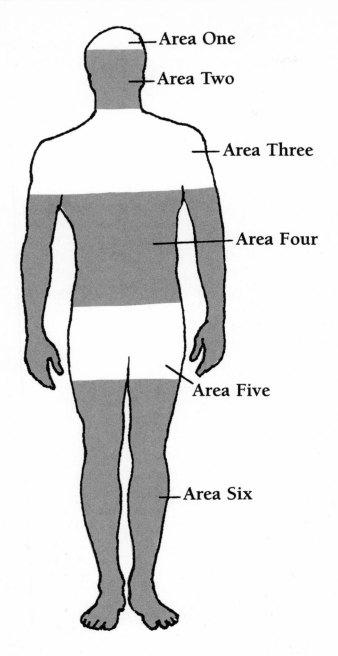

— Area One

— Area Two

— Area Three

— Area Four

— Area Five

— Area Six

ILLUS. 9 Safe Areas and No-Go Areas for Standing

temporarily support the weight of an average-sized woman. Make sure the back of his head is flat on the floor before you step up, and not tilted back. Also, he must hold his head still. I would recommend stepping up with one foot on his chest first, then carefully placing the other foot on his forehead. Or, if you have the proper support for your weight, stand with both feet on his forehead—briefly and carefully!

Next is Area Three and the sternum. The sternum is a strong bone and can support your weight temporarily. You will need to hold on to a door frame, or even the back of a sofa, to maintain your balance and keep your full weight off of him as you step up. A chin-up bar is useful as a support, also. Stand on his chest, facing him, and look down into his eyes. Gently, lift your feet up and down, like you are marching. Talk about standing on him in a sexy voice. Slowly squat down, then caress his face with your hand. This always drives the slave wild. Caution: *Do not step on his shoulders or below his nipples.*

Area Five is his hips and they should be stood on simultaneously (your chin-up bar will come in very handy here, too) to prevent injury. His genitals are in Area Five and are a wonderful place for a stroll but are obviously unable to support any weight. What you do to walk on his genitals is to stand somewhere else, like his sternum, and rock back and forth, shifting your weight from one to the other, alternating the pressure between the two areas. If he is also into humiliation, genital walking will be right up his alley.

If you are unable to install a chin-up bar in a doorway, you could use a door frame for support. This is acceptable since it will give you "a hand" but it doesn't give you much mobility if you want to walk up and down his body. You will not be able to walk hanging on to the door frame, so if you want to step on one area then another, you will have to step off him, have him move and then you can climb back on. This can be very distracting and break the mood as he squirms back and forth on the floor to reposition himself.

Now, let's talk about footwear for slave walking. I usually do the stroll in my stockinged feet or in a slightly lower heel than I would normally wear for such a session. Why a lower heel? Many men do not like to have a stiletto heel digging into them for more than a second or two. The higher the heel, the more you depend on the heel to distribute your weight, and the less you are able to stand on tippy toe (since you already are on tippy toe) and prevent the heel from digging into him. Some slaves do enjoy this greatly but your man is a beginner and a gaping chest wound might turn him off to further walking sessions.

My foot slaves have preferred the stockinged foot walk to the shod walk because it is more sensual and your toes are free to tease him. Try standing on his sternum and dipping one foot in and out of his mouth, talking to him the whole time about what a nice rug he makes or how cute he looks with your foot in his mouth or whatever diatribe he is partial to.

If you have no interest in a chin-up bar, and the door frame proves unsatisfactory for support, you can walk, or dance, on him in another way. I sit on edge of the sofa or my throne and have my slave lie perpendicular to it. When he has positioned himself, I support myself by my arms, keeping my buttocks off the sofa, and "walk" up and down his prone body. To "dance" up and down his body, I put on appropriate music and do a little dance on him as he lies there. Dancing in this manner is a lot of fun because you can do kick-ball chains (a jazz step) and fancy footwork you probably couldn't do even with the assistance of a chin-up bar. Since you are not really standing on him with your full weight, these two methods can also be used if he finds your weight on him too much to bear. This is also a wonderful method of genital walking as no real weight is put on his jewels. And remember, walking is a fine form of exercise!

A Sniffer's Story

One of my slaves is particularly enamored of sniffing my feet and shoes but does not want it to happen in a straightforward way. He wants to be "tricked" into it in several different ways. His favorite scenario is that I am the owner of the company he works for and I have received several complaints from his female superior about his lack of cooperation and outright insubordination. She asks me to have a chat with him to see if I can adjust his attitude.

I call him into my office after hours to discuss his situation. Finding him and his attitude of superiority unbearable (he can't understand why a woman is in a position of power and not he), I shove him under my desk and use him as a foot rest. I dangle my shoe off the end of my foot and when it falls off, I make him pick it up and replace it on my foot. But not before I make him read me the label inside. He protests that he is much too good to be "used" in such a manner, at which point, I take him by the back of his head and mash his face into my foot, berating him the whole time. I give him examples of a woman's superiority, internal plumbing, superior powers of organization, the ability to have children and propagate the race, rough draft (men) before the final masterpiece (women), and so on. He still protests that since he has a cock, he is superior. Then I slap his face several times and tie my pump to it (heel to his forehead). I demand that he sniff my shoe loud enough for me to hear it in spite of the pump muffling the sound. I order him to crawl on all fours after me as I walk down the hall, kissing each piece of carpet where I have stepped. For the grand finale, I walk on him, then stick one foot in his mouth, while covering his eyes with the other and verbally humiliating him at the same time. When he admits that women are superior to men in every way, I allow him to relieve himself in front me as his reward.

Shoe Fetishists and Shoe Worship

Although the foot fetishist certainly appreciates a nice shoe, the object of desire is still the foot. A shoe fetish is a fetish for the article itself. Women and men have shoe fetishes but the nature of the fetish varies. I am a shoe fetishist but I have no desire to lick the sole of my pumps or to suck on my heel. My desire is to possess as many pairs of beautiful shoes as I can stuff into the closet, many of which I will never wear out of the house. I am a classic example of a woman shoe fetishist.

Not sure if you have a shoe fetish? Let's make this really easy. Were you jealous of Imelda Marcos's shoe collection? Did you sympathize with the bartenderess who, upon winning the Lotto, ran off to buy "those red shoes" she wanted? Are you *always* shopping for shoes? Do you buy shoes for no apparent reason? Do you buy shoes first, then build an outfit around them? Have you ever bought a pair of shoes just because you have to have them? Do you have shoes that have been in your closet, unworn, since the day you brought them home?

Even one Yes answer qualifies you as a shoe fetishist. A fetishist of a mild degree but a fetishist all the same. Welcome to the club. I have never in my whole life met a woman who did not have a "thing" for shoes, even to a small degree.

Please do not use me as a role model in this area. I am telling you here and now that I am not rational when it comes to shoes. I buy shoes simply because I cannot leave the store without them. When I find a high-heeled pump that works for me, I buy several pairs in all the black hides it's made in. Occasionally, an exceptional pair of pumps in red or purple or green will catch my eye and I add them to my ever expanding collection. Then, I horde them against a dry spell (when no one is carrying styles I like) and break them out of storage when famine hits.

Naturally, the maintenance of my shoes is very important to me. Pumps frequently get new heels to keep up their appearance. My foot slave polishes them for me under my strictest supervision. An ordinary infraction earns him ten lashes. Inadequate buffing of my shoes earns him twenty! And heaven help him if he gets shoe polish on my foot.

I will say, in my own defense, that I have a terrible time getting shoes that fit properly. And I no longer buy a shoe hoping that I can "break it in." So a lot of my shoe shopping time is futile since I come home empty-handed. I shop for shoes more often than I buy them. Which always gives me something to do on Saturday afternoon.

The Tale of a Shoe Salesman

One afternoon, two of my girlfriends and I had lunch at a local bar and eatery. On the way there, we passed a shoe store. Of course, all three of us stopped to look in the window. And of course, I saw something I liked in the window and wanted to go in on the spot. My friends were hungry and promised to accompany me into the store after we ate. Knowing they weren't as crazed about shoes as I am, I really tried not to rush them through lunch just so I could indulge my fetish. Lunch drew to its inevitable close and I was the first one out of the restaurant.

And the first one into the shoe store. Pointing to the pumps of my desire, I called to the salesman for an eight and a half. Being winter, I was wearing big thick socks and cloddy boots to keep my tootsies warm and dry. The salesman came back with the shoes and I asked him for a ped, or footie. You can't try on pumps wearing socks. He came back with the peds, dropped them off, and went to stand by the register.

I kicked off the clodhoppers and stripped off the socks in short order, practically drooling to get my foot into these lovely shoes. As soon as my bare foot was exposed, the salesman literally flew to my side, then to my astonishment and amusement, dropped to his knees in front of me. When he had composed himself to speak, all he could say was, "Oh, you have the most beautiful feet. Slender, white-skinned, narrow, no corns, no bunions, no callouses. And delicious red polish on your lovely toes." Now it was his turn to drool and he looked torn with indecision when I suggested he put the shoe on my foot. He wanted me to buy the shoes and I had to try them on to do that, yet he was disappointed that the object of his desire was going to disappear into the pumps. A real dilemma for a foot fetishist shoe salesman.

The salesgirl must have seen and heard this before (I dubbed his performance "A Shoe Salesman's Ode to Feet") because she was standing there trying not to laugh and not succeeding. My girlfriends were highly amused by his obvious adoration, especially when he crawled over to the mirror I was admiring myself in and used his sleeve to buff away an imaginary scuff!

Well, I did buy those pumps, in black suede and black patent leather, and was most enthusiastically invited back to his store "anytime." Yes, thank you, and I'll be sure to have my feet with me when I do.

My favorite doorman, the one I found playing with the handcuffs, the same one who calls me on the intercom to tell me my cross-dressing friend looked "lovely" on a particular night, is also very observant when it comes to shoes. One evening when this doorman was on duty, I was returning home from dinner out with a friend, wearing a pair of delicious black knee boots that had been complaining of being in the closet unworn for, oh, years now. After we said good night, I crossed the lobby and headed for the stairs. As I hit the bottom step, I heard an appreciative "hmmmm" from the doorman. I turned to him, in a teasing voice, what the "hmmmm" meant. His response, "beautiful boots, Claudia, very sexy."

Now that we have ascertained that there are shoe fetishists lurking everywhere, what do you do if your man happens to be one of them?

As I just mentioned, the routine care and maintenance of your shoes and boots is an excellent task, but that should happen on a more or less daily basis. During a session, you want some special task for him to perform. He could give the bottom of your shoes a tongue bath. When I did this with my slave, I selected a pair of shoes that hadn't been worn outside but were scuffed and dusty from inside wear. (Some advanced fetishists purport to like cleaning a sole dirty from the street but I doubt that your mate will be one of them.) First I make myself comfortable then I cross my legs. I direct him to position himself under my dangling foot and perform whatever contortions necessary to reach my sole. Then the tongue bath begins. And I want to feel it through the leather sole of the shoe!

Tying One On

Foot worshipers who are also into humiliation just love to have your shoe, preferably your pump, tied to their face and/or their genitals. You'll need a slender rope from your bondage kit or a nice, long scarf. Two, if you'll be tying on two shoes. To tie the shoe to his face, place his chin in the toe of the shoe. His nose should be pushed into the instep with the heel of the pump extended over his forehead. Now loop your scarf or rope around the heel twice. Then taking the ends of the rope in either hand, pass each on top of his ears and around the back of his head. Cross them in back and pull the excess to the front. Retie. Continue until all the rope or scarf is used up and the shoe secured to his face. To tie the shoe to his genitals, stuff his sac into the heel and his cock into the toe. Use your second scarf or rope to secure it by looping it twice around the heel of the shoe then around his waist.

A great favorite of mine, since it is fun for me and humiliating for him, is to command him to give the heel of your shoe "head." This command always stuns them the first time! I favor a position similar to the one above for tongue cleaning. Again, I cross my legs, right over left. My slave then lies down with his head under my right foot. I "dip" my heel in and out of his mouth, slowly working it deeper down his throat. I take great care not to scrape his throat with my steel spike but before we are through, he *will* take the whole five inches.

Then I exhort him to suck, to suck my heel like he exhorted forgotten lovers of the past to suck his cock. He remembers that, doesn't
he? But that was a lifetime ago and he is another person now. That is
why he is yours, that is why you own him.

The Dangle

Since the dangle is neither the unshod foot or the shod foot but falls
halfway in between both, I thought a paragraph or two of its own would
be nice. The dangle is an art form of its own in the foot world. Most
successful when done with a pump, various mules also can be successfully dangled to the delight of the hypnotized beholder.

This is how the dangle is done. Cross your leg. Curl your foot in
your pump until the heel of your shoe pops off your foot. Now play
with the shoe as it hangs from your toes. Flick it fast, flick it slow, wiggle it left and right, pop it against your heel. See how many toes you
can take out without dropping it. Watch his eyes and head follow it in
its arcs and whirls. Is she going to drop it, he wonders. Then you flip
it and catch it and shake it back onto your foot. He will be watching
this in open-mouthed fascination, almost drooling I assure you. He will
become mesmerized by your foot and its toy shoe, playing like dolphins
together just out of his reach!

~ 9 ~

Humiliation and Head Games

As you have surmised by now, many fantasies include elements of other fantasies. Like a Chinese menu, some cross-dressers also like to be humiliated at the same time, foot worship merges with discipline, and bondage and discipline are like a hand in a glove. Humiliation comes in many forms and crosses many boundaries. It can take the form of a bare-bottomed over-the-knee (OTK) spanking or a ritual shaving off of his body hair. Humiliation is the dominant exerting her power over the submissive. By accepting the surrender of her submissive, the domina is elevated to a pedestal and honor is conferred upon her as if she were one of the aristocracy. Which she is. The submissive takes pride in his mistress's rank and is empowered by her power. Hence, his foot kissing, kneeling, wearing her collar and leash, and other signs of homage are not degrading to the slave but are acts performed in pride. He is proud of his mistress and her ability to train him, proud to be owned by such a powerful mistress.

Verbal Humiliation

Your slave may tell you that he wants you to verbally humiliate him. You are hesitant at first. But humiliating him (or embarrassing him) and degrading him are two different things. Erotic verbal humiliation may be an important part of his fantasy and provide a safe outlet for those fantasies. If done well, a good head game can be as satisfying as a physical act. In D&S, humiliation often builds the individual up, not tears them down. This can involve taking inhibitions and trucking them out into the light and turning them upside down. But this is not a mind fuck. Although you are making him do something that will make him look or feel silly, the excitement comes from his compliance and cooperation.

"Dirty talk" is a very common form of verbal abuse that few think of as humiliation. Name-calling is a popular form of dirty talk. Your "hero" by day turns into your "worm" at night. A quiet type by day, he may become your "slut" by night. Many also find it exciting to have their partner call their body parts by slangy or insulting names. During the day, he could have a nice round bottom; at night; a juicy ass for beating. Maybe you do this already; many otherwise vanilla couples indulge in this kind of play. Humiliation like this is not for everyone. This is an area which should be discussed carefully if he tells you verbal humiliation is one of his buttons. You don't want to say the wrong thing and leave him feeling degraded or abused. Humiliation as a D&S practice should have prior and clear consent by both partners. This is where communication beforehand is extremely important. D&Sers agree that head games are very complex and that a good, sensitive D&S head game can create an emotional bond between the two of you. Since he won't be asking you to scold or berate or humiliate a genuine flaw in his character, he is free to experience his fantasy. Being scolded for being highly sexed is a popular humiliation fantasy. Whether or not he is highly sexed is immaterial, being scolded for being a slut is thrilling.

The best scenario, of course, would be for him to tell you the object of his humiliation. Perhaps he wants you to belittle his genitals. Or tell him he is not worthy to serve you, or lick your shoes, or breathe the same air. He may want you to call him promiscuous, a little slut, anyone's for the asking. Or he may like being told that he'll be given to your friends to "service" them when they need it.

He may have a "trigger" word or phrase, like "baby" or "just wait till I get you home." If you watch him closely each time you say the word or phrase, you will see there is a specific reaction to it. A certain glazed look in his eyes, an audible intake of breath and, hopefully, a hardening of his cock.

His taste in verbal humiliation can also include his humiliating himself. He may prefer to belittle himself on your command, rather than have you say it. If this is his fantasy, you can set it up by discussing beforehand what he is going to say about himself. Then you can prompt him to make the "proper" responses. A popular turn-on phrase is "I am your slave, Mistress." It excites him to call himself a slave. So you may elicit this response by asking him who he belongs to or what he is.

Others want only to be threatened with humiliation or a humiliating punishment. If he has a chest hair arrangement that he is particularly proud of, threaten to shave it off if he doesn't obey. If cross-dressing is not his desire, threaten to dress him up *and* take him out. You can be wonderfully creative with this fantasy and show him how lucky he is to have a mistress who is so imaginative!

Another popular request is for you to ask him who his cock belongs to. "Is this my cock?" you ask him in a sweet, sexy tone. "Yes, Mistress," is his response. Then in a slightly sterner tone, ask him the same question. His response will be the same. Let's assume at this point that his hard-on isn't all you want it to be. Repeat your question for the third time and after he answers, hit it gently with your hand, or whip, and in your best mistress voice demand to know why, if it's yours, it isn't hard. Make him stroke himself in front of you until you are satisfied with the results.

How Big Was It?

One evening I saw a client, a pleasant young man who wanted me to verbally humiliate him. This was unusual because this type of D&S is best done by and with someone who knows you well to really make it work. But he did tell me the manner in which he wanted to be humiliated and I made my preparations. I arrived at the house (of domination) before he did and set myself up in the dungeon. He knocked and I gave him permission to enter. As he entered the room, his eyes widened in surprise, he gasped, "Oh!" and quickly put his head down. I was arranged in the leather chair I used as my throne, wearing a very sexy leather teddy, opera length leather gloves, thigh-high stockings and over-the-knee boots. Around my hips I had my harness and attached to that, my strap-on! I was sitting there on my throne, stroking this huge dildo just like it was a real erection and it was mine! Some of this was prearranged: I knew his fantasy was to be verbally humiliated by a woman whose "genitals" where bigger than his and that I could say pretty much what I wanted in that context. Hence, the harness and strap-on and the leather teddy, tough but still sexy.

I ordered him to stand and undress for me (in the order I prefer) telling him we would at least go through the motions since he was here but . . . no man really had genitals big enough to satisfy me. When he dropped his boxers, I dropped my jaw. Let me stress that I had chosen a sizable dildo, a good nine inches long and almost two inches thick, for his fantasy. It was one of the largest ones I had that was still realistic. There's no other way to say it: his own equipment put my fake stuff to shame! To shame! I was unclear as to how it all fit in his shorts! Clearly, he had to have it taped to his leg at some point to stop the thing from dragging on the ground.

I wondered if he was joking: one of those terrible subs who fight and test the mistress's authority at every opportunity. But when I looked at his face, I saw that he was serious. No glint of humor twinkled in his eyes nor crinkling in the corners of his mouth, like a smile held in. So I took him at face value and tried to go on. Since both of us could see that his was bigger than mine, belittling its littleness wasn't going to work. But it *was* bent off to the left whereas *mine* was perfectly and beautifully straight. So I went to "work" starting with that: "Look at that! Why is it *bent* like that? Mine is so nice and straight. Do you think you'll ever be able to put that bent thing inside of anyone, anyone at all? Who would want it? Bent as it is!" This line of humiliation seemed to do it for him because the thing continued to grow to gargantuan proportions right before my eyes.

Normally this type of humiliation would be more satisfying from someone you are in a relationship with because this foundation can be added to, built on to incorporate more of his and your fantasies.

Humiliation fantasies vary as much from person to person as everything else does, but the fantasy of exposing oneself to another, or many others, is a favorite scenario. In a private setting, this can be a moving experience for the new sub since it may well be the first time he has ever been so exposed to the gaze of another. The exposure, of course, involves his genitals and a humiliating position. One position favored for this is to have him kneel on the bed, feet and knees wide apart. Next he is to bend forward until his head and shoulders touch the bed. Then instruct him to raise his hips. See what this does to him. By now he is probably panting into the coverlet or duvet and his erection is starting. Now instruct him to reach back and spread his cheeks. The cheeks of his butt. Step around and make it clear that you are inspecting him. Make your eyes so hot he can feel their heat when you look at him, or look him over. He feels like an object on display, asked to turn this way and that before being assessed and bought, or rejected.

Last-Minute Humiliation

One evening I had a date with a man; a tall, rich man in his early forties. We had been introduced over the phone by a mutual friend and after a dozen phone conversations, we decided to meet. He described himself to me as being tall (he was) red haired (where he had hair, it was red) and very attractive (to his mother). I'm sure some women found him attractive for himself and I'm equally sure that all those millions in the bank and the palatial mansion in the Hamptons added to his allure. I didn't find him to be handsome and since I've never been attracted to the size of a man's wallet (until recently!), I wasn't particularly interested in his money.

But we did make a date and I decided to see it through. He was parading around his lovely apartment as proud as a rooster in a hen house and making a pompous ass out of himself in the process. He pointed out common objects to me as if I had never seen a fireplace or dining room. We were supposed to have dinner but he had eaten before I arrived. His solution was to serve me a catered dinner set up on a folding tray table in the living room. I ate alone as he watched me. How awkward! How rude! I gritted my teeth and bore it; it would be over soon anyway.

The whole purpose of my being there was to practice my caning on him. He was a masochist, not a submissive. We had discussed this thoroughly on the phone for quite some time a few days prior to my arrival. He disrobed at my command, put his clothes out of sight and stood before me for my inspection. I was horrified! His buttocks were covered in cane marks! And there, right across the center of his member, was another big ugly bruise.

"What happened here? Where did you got those?" I inquired, not bothering to keep the disgust out of my voice. "I was so excited by our conversations that I couldn't wait. Just last night I hired someone else to come give me a caning," was his idiotic answer. And I really was disgusted with him. Disgusted because he couldn't control himself to wait one more night for my arrival, disgusted because instead of a blank "canvas" on which to paint my strokes, the surface was marred by someone else's handiwork. Disgusted because he had paid someone else to make a mess of his ass when he wasn't paying me. And disgusted because he was so proud of himself and his marks that he wasn't even sensitive enough to discern that I was unhappy with the present situation.

I gave him a half-hearted caning, very disappointed that I couldn't tell my marks from the ones left by the previous night's session. He was so selfish he didn't even notice that my heart wasn't in what I was doing. I packed up my equipment and got ready to go.

As I got ready to leave he popped the question.

"So, what do you think? Am I everything I said I was?" He asked in his European accent. I said to myself, you asked for it, mister. I hope you can take it. "First," I said, "those marks you presented me with really turned me off. You knew I was coming and you couldn't control yourself for one more night until my arrival? As far as your physical aspects are concerned, you are tall, I'll give you that. But handsome? You are not my idea of handsome. As a matter of fact, I was so disappointed when you opened the door, I almost left!"

Although I had caned him earlier in the evening, this was much more painful and humiliating for him. All that money assured him he would never be rejected—he was accustomed to doing the rejecting. Here was this almost dainty woman (so poor she had to take the bus home) doing exactly that! Ask me if it felt good and I'll tell you, unequivocally, Yes!

Public Humiliation

What, you may be saying, is public humiliation and why would anyone be interested in it? Last things first. Public humiliation is a fascinating subject and one with deep psychological implications. We are not going to deal with the heavy psychological stuff here—I am not qualified to do so and such things can be so subjective, and vary so much from one individual to the next, that generalizations are almost useless.

Public humiliation is not to everyone's taste and most men who enjoy public humiliation are specific about their preferences. Their preferences can run the gamut from being handcuffed to a park bench and asking total strangers to unlock them to being humiliated in front of one person only. A favorite in the "mild" area is to be verbally humiliated in front of a total stranger.

One gentleman with a high-powered position literally terrorized his employees. These poor people quaked in fear of him, especially the secretaries (sound like anyone you know?). One evening, he asked me out to dinner and requested that I plan something special to humiliate him. And this is a popular one with the mistresses. All of us seem to know it but it's always new to the men.

I met him outside the restaurant, a macho-type steak and chop house on Fourteenth Street and Ninth Avenue in Manhattan. I was a few minutes late, of course (better that he wait for me rather than I for him). I demanded that he give me his wallet and all of his money. He got very excited when I ordered him to hand it over but then seemed puzzled that nothing else was forthcoming. When I was satisfied that I had custody of every last cent in his pockets and all of his plastic, we went inside and were seated.

We spent the meal making small talk, led by me. I was very careful not to let the conversation stray toward what I had planned for him. I wanted him to think that relieving him of his money was all I could dream up. Ha!

After we had finished dining, the waiter predictably presented my male companion with the check. This was when I executed my plan. In a sweet singsong tone, I said to the waiter, "Give the check to me. I don't allow him to have any money of his own." My companion's jaw dropped and then snapped shut as he hung his head in shame. The waiter recovered his aplomb quickly and smilingly handed me the check.

As you can see, this was mild since only one person witnessed it yet it was still public. My companion was very satisfied with this little drama, especially since the dinner had been so normal in all other respects and I had saved the best for last.

If you are fortunate enough to have some friends who indulge in D&S, you can create all sorts of scenarios to publicly humiliate the slaves in your group. And you can do it in your own home, too.

If he is a foot worshiper and a slave at your hen party, assign him the duty of massaging feet on demand. Or he could shine your guests' shoes or act as an ottoman or hassock. At the end of the evening, have each lady critique his performance (à la Annabella) and discipline him for his infractions. A favorite is to have him wear one of your undergarments, usually panties, to work under his regular business clothes. No one will actually *see* them (you can be sure he'll be using a stall that day), but he will be aware of them all day. Each time he moves, their unaccustomed silkiness will caress his skin. They will bunch in strange places. And he will have to keep reminding himself that there is no flap or opening in the front and they must be pulled down. You will be on his mind all day. The unpredictable mind of the mistress is part of what makes D&S so enjoyable for both of you.

Objectification/Depersonalization

The term "depersonalization" is new to me but I feel it is also so descriptive of what I call "objectification" that I will include it here as being one and the same state. Objectification fantasies revolve around the slave becoming something less than human: an animal or an inanimate object, or a sex toy being the most popular. In the "Foot Fetishes" chapter, there is a cat scenario that would fulfill an animal objectification fantasy nicely. In the inanimate object department, a footstool or footrest, a piece of artwork, a table base or other piece of furniture, and an ashtray seem to be the front runners. As for the sex toy fantasy . . . well, who hasn't had one of those?

For the dominant, objectification will be fun for those who enjoy exerting tight control over their slaves. When you ignore his personality and treat him like a thing with no thoughts or feelings, he experiences the total subjugation of his will to yours and can enjoy his powerlessness guiltlessly. When I have trained slaves to be objects they have reported to me feelings of extreme peace and calm. One said, "When I am my mistress's footstool, I cease to think of the world outside, the beeper, the cell phone. My sole purpose is to cushion my lady's feet and knowing that, my mind is free. It is part of the dynamics of my surrender to her that I be so totally in her power that she can do anything to me, make me into anything, turn me to any use." For the submissive, objectification can fulfill many a humiliation fantasy that crystallizes the slave's sexual excitement.

In the D&S world, thousands enact scenes where the submissive is "forced" or coerced into living out his fantasies. This is done with his full cooperation, and in tandem with the dominant partner. The consent and coercion scenario makes thousands achieve multiple orgasms, sometimes on command.

Objectification is considered by some D&Sers to be "dangerous ground" because of the possible deep psychological aspects of the game. As you are probably playing with a long-standing partner, with proper communication, I don't see this as being a problem. I have had slaves furnish entire rooms for me; I have been a footstool myself. It is hard work being the dominant and to take a moment and put your feet up . . . ah! And a good slave will realize how hard you are working to give him his pleasure and be happy to accommodate you as your footstool.

I loved to train slaves to be objects, to be still and motionless, and to try to become the object they are imitating. To be a truly good object, the slave must be able to enter a very special space, sometimes called "sub space" or sometimes just referred to as "going under." I know many of my slaves have attained true objectification. What both of these terms mean is a state of mind that the sub enters when the dominant has touched a cord in the sub and a deep connection has been made. In sub space, all that exists for the sub is the dominant. The sound of the dominant's voice, the dominant's touch and the dominant's strength are all that connect the submissive to Planet Earth. With an invisible umbilical cord, the top is connected to the bottom and anchors the bottom to this world so the bottom is free to explore and experience new heights of sexuality and sensuality. The dominant protects the sub and the sub trusts implicitly in the dom's ability to do this.

Some dominants disdain objectification, but I don't see what all the fuss is about. They say it is too passive and they like to have a sub who's more lively. They seem to forget that the object doesn't remain an object forever—just for a short time. This would only be a consideration if he *really* did turn into footstool! To give the dom a break, to humble the sub for an infraction or for importuning, to break his pride—objectification is good for all this. For the sub who likes to give, who has a nurturing spirit, objectification is a gift of selflessness to the dom. It tells the dom, "Don't think about me for a while, stop entertaining me. You look tired, put your feet up." Then the sub assumes the footstool position most favored by the dom and offers his back or his belly or his buttocks for the dom's comfort.

Pony Boys and Pony Girls

Pony boys and pony girls deserve a few lines of their own because their fetish requires such time and devotion and physical stamina. My first exposure to ponies was in the *Beauty Trilogy*, by Anne Rice writing as A. N. Roquelaure (see "Recommended Reading" for particulars). Rice's ponies were all male, and their exotic and humiliating training fascinated me. Naked, shod with pony boots with hooves, plugs with streaming horsetails protruding from their asses, bitted, reined and harnessed, pony boys transported young and old, rich and poor through the streets of the village. Eating and sleeping in the stables and used by the grooms, the life of a pony boy was one of all body and no mind. Wouldn't that be nice once in a while?

But if you were a woman, a mere five years ago the "pony" fantasy was just that. A practical cart was still a fantasy, as women are unable to support the weight of a man on their backs. So their training consisted of mostly prancing and gaits and looking good in a pony outfit. Then someone built a cart for the ponies to pull and voila! Whereas one pony girl cannot carry a man, one could pull a cart with a man in it. Two or three ponies would pull it faster and longer. The pony girl became a reality.

Some ponies are only trained to the rein and others are trained to provide more tangible service to their masters. Working ponies are usually outfitted by their mistress/trainer in boots, leather thongs, and chest harnesses. Arms bound in leather behind their backs, corsets snug, bits in their mouths, pony girls in stilettos high step in sync to pull the cart smoothly and in tandem. Their plumed headdresses quiver erotically with each step as they draw their lord implacably forward.

Carts and rigs vary from the short and squat wheelbarrow variety for two or more ponies to the high-seated, spidery-wheeled remade rickshaw for one pony and one rider to Master Keith's elegant chariot drawn by three beautiful pony girls. In "Designersex," the video from the 1995 Rubber Ball, sponsored by Skin Two of London (see "Shopping Guide" for address), there are two beautifully and erotically filmed segments of Master Keith outfitting his three pony girls followed by some very sexy footage of the ponies drawing the cart.

~ 10 ~

Party Games

Party Games is an unusual chapter for a beginner's guide to D&S but the games are so much fun, I couldn't keep them to myself. Some of the games we'll talk about are old favorites reworked to have a D&S theme; others I made up myself when I was throwing scene parties.

The secret of any memorable party is good food, good friends, and good times. The food and friends are easy but it is up to the hostess/mistress to provide the good times. There is more to a successful party than just eating and drinking. When the food is finished, you must have something in mind for your guests to do. This is especially helpful when the group you have invited is a mix of people who don't know everyone else and tend to stick with the people who they came with, or already know. A lack of mingling ensues as cliques form and splinter off. The best way to prevent this from happening is to plan out a game you want your guests to play. How do you induce everyone to play the game? You bribe them, of course! Having a little party favor to give to each of them for their role in the festivities will persuade them to get up and play.

First make a list of all your guests. Unless you have a lot of discretionary income, if you have more than fifteen to twenty guests, you may want to make "awards" for best costume or best trained slave, rather than gift each guest. Then, pen in hand, stop and consider each person on the list. Think about what that person enjoys, or what their hobby or disposition is (foot slave, stern disciplinarian, "top" or "bottom") and decide if you would like to get them a funny party favor or a practical one. Since this is supposed to be a D&S party, the party favors should be of a D&S nature and reflect the tastes of your guests.

Here are some of my favorite picks to give out as party favors and an idea of what each one will cost you in the New York City area:

For The Mistresses: A long plumelike feather ($5) available at millinery supply shops, whip key chain ($4), sleep mask ($6 to $10), universal handcuff key ($6), sheer black stockings ($2 to $4), riding crop ($12), candle in a tall glass ($4), five hardware-store rubber O-rings in graduating sizes (under $1 each, for cock bondage), small whips ($10), thick wooden ruler ($2).

For The Slaves: handcuff tie tack ($5), handcuff pierced earring ($5 to $6 for one), body fingerpaints ($8), lollipop condoms and individual one-shot lubricants (under $2 for both), massage oil (to use on her, under $10), pedicure supplies like a callous remover ($3) or nail brush ($2).

For Either: leather and silver studded mistress/slave bracelets ($6 to $10), chain choke collar from the pet shop ($8 to $12), a pair of six- or nine-foot black buckskin laces ($4 for both), spray bottle of latex polish ($8).

And of course, you can give the same gift, like the universal handcuff key, to a couple of different guests to save yourself some extra running around. Or the lollipop condom/one-shot lube can be given to each male guest.

Now that you have spent all this time and money on shopping for these things, and then more time wrapping them, you may be asking yourself (or me) what's in it for me? Lots of things, in no particular order. You acquire a "name" for having great parties and everyone wants to be invited; your guests have a great time and show their appreciation on your birthday; you get to control the action, excuse me, the *festivities*; you get to be the star of your own show; you can take lots of great pictures to look at in your old age and keep yourself young-minded. If you picked "control the action" as your first reason for having a D&S party, you are in luck. Since it is also my main reason, and the reason for all those party favors, I am going to talk about it next.

It has been my experience at small parties that it starts to get going about an hour after the last guests have arrived. About an hour after that is when small cliques begin to form, and the newcomers get left out. This is your time to gather everyone together around you and announce your plans to play a game. Some will be hesitant or dismissive. And this is where those favors come out. You go on to tell your guests that there will be a prize for the winners, or everyone, for participating in the game. Who doesn't want a prize? Or a gift? And your mistresses/girlfriends will help prod their slaves into it.

Indoor Games

The Basket Of Doom

This is my personal favorite. It is best for a small group of fifteen to twenty, made up of mostly D&S players. Each person picks a slip of paper from a basket and does whatever is written on it to receive their prize. These "commands" could range from performing "I'm a Little Tea Pot" and "Walking Like an Egyptian", for those new to the scene, to foot worship and fetching the ball, for those who are not.

In the first variation of this game, only slaves pick from the basket. The mistresses give a small display of their specialty and are gifted after their "performance." A nice touch is to have your slave crawl to the mistress and present her with her gift.

The second variation on "the Basket of Doom" is to have two baskets, one for slaves and one for mistresses, and everyone picks from their basket. The commands to the Mistress could include a flogging demonstration or walking the "dog", either her own or someone else's. To play either variation of this game, you obviously must have a prize or gift for everyone.

Mistress Says

For a group that is not made up of entirely D&S players, or at least ones accepting of it, "Mistress Says" is my recommendation. If your mate is assisting you with hosting (and he damn well should be), he can help you think up things for your guests that are appropriate for them to do to "earn" their prize.

I'll give you some examples of things I had my guests do at one of my parties. Everyone was into D&S on some level but some were new to it and shy about doing a scene "in public." So we had to gear each performance to fit the couple.

I asked one couple to dirty dance together and, getting Roman thumbs up or down from the other guests, they couldn't stop until all of us were satisfied. My co-host, another dominant but under my direction, presented the gifts.

An experienced foot slave was made to worship his inexperienced young mistress's feet. One couple was made up of a dominant woman and submissive male with loads of experience. He was made to give her a pony ride back and forth across the room, being cropped all the way.

Those are some different level activities for your guests to do. The game also takes up a lot of time since each couple has to perform, then wants to open their gifts right away. By the time the game is over, your guests will have had such a great time that they will go home shortly thereafter. "It's three-thirty? Wow! We have to get going."

Musical Chairs

Another fun game for a mixed group is "Musical Chairs." In regular Musical Chairs, there is one less chair than there are players. In this variation, say there are twenty players; you would use nineteen chairs. Two people are expected to sit in one chair; the slave on the bottom and the mistress on top of him. The slave who doesn't get a chair and therefore leaves the mistress unseated can be made to do one of two things: He could be punished as in the game "Old Mill," where, at the end of the game, the winners lined up with their legs open far enough part for the disgraced one to crawl between them. As he crawled through, the winner standing above him paddled his fanny as he went by. D&S players call this very game "Running the Gauntlet." The bad slave is made to run through a gauntlet made up of mistresses with their implement of choice.

Or you can borrow the Basket of Doom, since only slaves will be losing, and have him do what he picks as his punishment. The last couple with a seat receives a prize.

In the second version, the regular rules apply: one rear end to a chair. The difference being that in this version the slaves themselves become the chairs. Start with ten mistresses and nine "chairs." The unseated mistress and one chair-slave is eliminated each time the music stops, leaving a mistress without a seat the next time the music stops. Now there are nine mistresses and eight chairs. And so on until there is only one chair left for the two mistresses. The mistress that wins the seat wins a prize.

"Slave Auction"

Holding a slave auction is a great way to entertain your guests; however, I would only recommend it for a small, intimate group because the highest bidder gets the slave. So you have to be sure that no one would object to having her slave bought by one lady or another and that no slave would object to a particular mistress.

This is not a permanent arrangement. It lasts for a couple of hours or the duration of the party and that's it. To play this game, no gifts are needed but you do have to have some sort of funny money to turn in on the purchase. Use large "bills," nothing less than hundreds, and go up to five hundred and thousand-dollar bills. The larger the denominations are, the more fun the auction becomes. You could use Monopoly money; or if you are creative, or have lots of time, you can make up your own money. You need to distribute the money unequally to your guests.

Here's one idea: Each mistress has a slave. Each mistress receives X number of dollars for every well-executed service her slave performs. If and when her slave screws up, she pays a fine to the offended mistress. This way, when bidding time comes, each mistress has a different amount of money and the bidding becomes more interesting. It is against the rules to bid on the slave you brought with you.

Now you need a way to make the mistresses bid on the slaves. As the mistress of ceremonies, you can opt for the ever-popular Basket of Doom. Or each mistress can write up a short spiel about her slave. As you read out each of his specialties, he has to give a little demonstration of it to the ladies. Then you invite the ladies to start the bidding at $500. And do the routine: "I have five, I have five, who'll give me six? Who'll give me six for this fine male slave? Six? I have six. Do I hear seven?" The slave should be hamming it up, trying to drive his bidding price higher, especially if he likes who is bidding on him. The ladies will be laughing at his antics and making their slaves run to do more tasks to earn them more money. With the right group, "Slave Auction" is a big hit and gets talked about for weeks afterwards.

This game has a hidden benefit for both the mistress and the slave. The mistress gets to test her skill and the limits of a slave she hasn't played with before. The slave gets to experience a new mistress's rules and expected level of service. This broadens your slave's horizons and increases his appreciation of you. During the swapping, both doms and subs often learn new things from their temporary partners and incorporate them into their own repertoire.

Outdoor Games

D&S Bar-B-Que? No problem! You have a willing and eager slave to help you with the chores and act as co-host. If he is handling the cooking fire, make sure he wears his undies or one of those big, silly chef's aprons to protect himself. And he should play an instrumental part in getting the other slaves organized to play the games you have planned for your guests. I am going to give you only three examples of outdoor games because almost any game can be turned into a D&S game.

Bareback Pony Races

One of my favorites, pony races can be played on dry land or in a pool, if you are lucky enough to have one. If on land, plot out a course for the ponies to follow—starting point, midpoint, and finish line. Each mistress's slave is her mount. You need not worry about saddles because I will describe to you how to stay on without one.

First, you will need a mounting stool (any sturdy chair or stepladder will do) and a crop of some sort. This is a race and your pony will need encouragement if you are to win. If someone is without a crop, and you live near trees, see if a slave can locate a thin, pliable, young branchlet and then strip it of its leaves. This should work well.

Next, mount your pony. The pony should be standing with his feet firmly planted about eighteen inches apart with his back end toward the mounting post. Have him bend his knees a little and tilt his upper body forward at about a thirty-degree angle. When he is ready, you should climb onto his lower back and wrap your legs around him. His hips will help keep you on him. When you are situated, he should hold on to your legs to help you stay there.

Now you need reins. If you don't have a bit, you really don't have anything to attach the reins to so I would recommend grabbing a handful of his hair and using that (just like you are riding bareback and you are holding on to the horse's mane to stay on). Since you are not really guiding him with the "reins" this should not be a problem for your pony. After all, he can still see where he is supposed to go and he can still hear your commands. If you are right-handed, hold on with the left to keep your right hand free for cropping him along. When you are mounted, move him over to the starting line.

When all the riders and their ponies are assembled, give the signal that the race has begun. You can clap your hands, blow a whistle, or pop a balloon. You can even yell, "They're off!" if you like.

If some of your guests are not participating, encourage them to cheer their favorite team on. Some friendly wagering by the mistresses for the services of their slaves would help to liven things up even more. The handier mistresses might want to make up numbers for each rider and pony, just like a real horse race. Or a finish line banner for the winning pony to break through. Lastly, you will need prizes for the winners and some sort of punishment for the losers.

Keeping with the horsey theme, you may want to consider roses for the winning mistress and a nice grooming for her mount. For the losers, the mistress of the last place pony could determine what punishment he will receive from the guests or she could punish him herself in front of the guests, of course. Or making him run the gauntlet is always nice.

Fetch

Although you can also play this game inside, I prefer outside in the yard because you have so much more room to throw the ball or stick he will be retrieving.

Fetch is pretty self-explanatory but there are a couple of variations on what your slave/dog does and how he does it. You could have him retrieve the ball on all fours like a real dog. If he has bad knees, or the yard is gravelly, he could be on two legs. I prefer on all fours.

You can take your choice of a ball or a stick. If you choose a stick, make sure it is clean and has no sharp things sticking out of it to hurt his mouth. I prefer a ball to a stick. Go into a pet shop and look at the dogs' fetching balls. Make sure it is small enough for him to pick up in his mouth. Dog's jaws open up considerably farther than ours so you may have to try it on for size in the pet shop. (I did, to the great amusement of the salesman.) Also, a ball can be washed with soap and water and stored for the next time.

Slave/dogs can be sneaky. It is certainly easier to pick the ball up in your hand and stick in your mouth than it is to pick it up in your mouth. If you don't watch him, he will try to place it in his teeth manually. Hit him with a rolled up newspaper and say, "No," in your best dominant/trainer tone.

Then make him fetch again. If he still picks it up in his hand, tie his leash to the leg of the table and don't let anyone play with him or other "dogs" come and sniff him.

Have your mistress friends line up with their dogs at their sides. Give a signal to throw the ball. The first slave back with the ball, or stick, in his teeth has won for his mistress. You should gift her with some small item from the list in the beginning of this chapter and reward the slave/dog by letting him do the thing he most desires. Kiss toes, massage feet, whatever his D&S preference is.

Ruffs

Ruffs can be played either indoors or out, with an unlimited number of people as long as half of them want to be dogs. Just the two of you or a dozen competing teams. Ruffs is fun. If you are going to play this game as a competition, you will need some people to sit out and be judges. If it is just the two of you, Ruffs is a very good training session.

If you have ever brought your dog to "obedience school," then you basically know how to play Ruffs. If you are new to the experience, here are a few things to think about before you begin. What commands will you teach him? Will you use the "word" or assign it a number? Many use numbers to stop strangers from giving commands to their pet. If you teach him that "one" means "sit," he won't become confused by strangers shouting "sit" at him. This is like your own secret language, just between you and your pet. He should be in his collar and on his leash in whatever state of dress of undress you have agreed on.

The first thing you may want to teach him is to "heel." This is usually a "word" command and not assigned a number. Heeling means that when you walk, his shoulder should remain against your leg and his pace and gait should match yours. When he heels, you gather the excess leash up in your hand. This keeps him from straying. In other words, when he heels, keep him on a short leash.

Next, you may want to consider teaching him to sit, which many call "one." Stay, or "two," which can also be followed by a hand sign, would be the next command. To perform the hand sign, bring the palm of your hand down and perpendicular to his nose in combination with the verbal command "stay!". "Three" or "down" could be his next command; four could mean "roll over." Five could be "beg"; six, or a loud smooching noise could be "come."

It is very easy to turn this into a party game. Each trainer/dog team can perform the pet's complete repertoire and then be scored by the judges. Or each team can compete in each event separately (the "sit" event, then the "beg" event), and the team with the highest total at the end wins.

All the best parties are made up of equal parts good company, good food, and good times. I hope this chapter has given you ideas for games and hostess gifts that make your parties a D&S success!

~ 11 ~

Positions

Positions are so interesting to me that I decided to devote a chapter to the different ones he can be trained to assume on command. "Positions" is not to be confused with "Mental Bondage" where the slave is told to assume and hold a certain position for a specified amount of time. "Positions," in all its varieties, is very different and a lot more fun for both of you.

I divide "Positions" into two separate categories. The first is positions that the slave can be trained to assume at the mistress's command. I call these the Training Positions. Ten in number, they include a greeting for the mistress, waiting and inspection positions, and confession and forgiveness positions, to name a few. Some are simply designed to keep him out of the way at a party or club. Training him in the proper execution of these positions can creatively entertain both of you for many hours of D&S play. An additional benefit is that he becomes accustomed to obeying one-word commands from you without hesitation. Training him to these positions should elevate his spirit; it should no more shame him to assume these positions at your whim than it would to kiss your shoe or draw breath. You should be like the Great Queen to him, the One to whom all others pay homage. To prostrate himself before you is an honor; to demonstrate these positions on command to show your expertise and control as a dominant is an honor; as a devoted slave he will want to perform with grace and obedience.

And if he doesn't, there are the second set of positions, Punishment Positions! Of course, there are hundreds of positions to punish him in and we're not going to describe them all here—just a few of my favorites for caning, spanking, and whipping! As you become more skilled, you can create your own positions, give them a number, and add them to his growing repertoire of trained positions.

Training Positions

Position One

Position One is my favorite and I am a stickler for its proper execution. It is the position for greeting the mistress and must be done with all the grace and devotion he can muster.

What you do: You may either sit or stand. If you are seated, you can cross your legs or simply extend one foot forward of the other; if you are standing, extend one foot slightly forward of the other. Now, look regal and deserving of the homage.

What he does: His eyes are downcast at all times. He drops to his knees as gracefully as he can and sits back on his heels momentarily. His butt should not stick out when he does this—it should be more like "sinking" down. (At this point, the tops of his feet are flat on the floor.) Next, he leans forward, his head and shoulders drop to the floor right in front of your extended foot and his hands are placed one on either side of the proffered foot. His feet and knees should not move when he leans forward. When he drops his head and shoulders to the floor, his hips should be up and his back held in a smooth, pleasing line. The fingers of his hands on either side of your foot should be closed and his hands flat to the floor. His elbows should be tucked in to his sides. Finally, he touches his forehead to the toe of your foot and waits for your signal.

As he performs each movement, watch his technique, or style if you prefer, and correct him as needed. Did his butt stick out on the initial prostration? Was his back in a pleasing line? Fingers closed? How was his attitude? Did he show the proper homage, the proper respect? Did he wait patiently for the next signal? Practice it with him until he performs it as smoothly as a dancer (we hope), reward him (or not, your choice) and teach him Position Two.

Position Two

Position Two is the position for a "standing inspection." And although it is an inspection position, there is no humiliation associated with it. It is the position for a slave who takes pride in his servitude and knows he is presenting his best self to the mistress for her inspection. His head is up; his eyes are straight ahead. The humiliation comes in with the variation, or subposition.

What you do, part one: He has just executed Position One and his head is on your foot, waiting for your signal. You can signal him by curling your toes inside your shoe or verbalize your acceptance by commanding to him assume another position. Then move on to the next phase.

What he does: He rises, again as gracefully as he can. The rise should be the exact opposite motion of the movement he performed to get down. It's all in the toes—ask any geisha girl! He steps back from you and spreads his feet about eighteen inches apart. Then: head up, eyes front, shoulders back, tummy tucked, hands clasped behind the neck, elbows out, arms parallel to the floor. And he awaits your pleasure.

What you do, part two: Walk around him, look him up and down. Make him feel your eyes on him as you inspect your property. Correct his stance, kick his feet apart, flatten his elbows, lift his chin. Satisfied? Now for the "variation."

Call out "hup" or whatever you have agreed upon to denote the variation or just say "bend" or "over" or "bend over," which is exactly what you want him to do. On command he is to bend at the waist, and here you have a choice: his hands can remain clasped behind his head, he can rest his hands on his knees with his elbows out, or he can grasp his ankles. But in any case, he is now exposed to your gaze and should be feeling the heat of it. Running your nails over his balls and your hand over a buttock cheek would be nice right now. Take your time. When you are through, a stinging little smack on the butt could signal that the inspection is over and he has been accepted, or to stand up straight. This is the humiliating variation on Position Two.

Position Three

Position Three is the "at-ease" position described in earlier chapters. This is a waiting position, as in waiting for your next command.

What you do: Call out "three" from whatever position you are comfortable in. It is a waiting position for him, not you!

What he does: He drops to his knees. (In my case, I prefer him slightly to the left of my feet so he doesn't get in my way or restrict my movement.) He rests his buttocks on his heels; the tops of his feet are flat to the floor, in other words, soles up. His knees are always open as his genitals are always to be available to you for your inspection and use; he rests his hands palms down on his thighs. His shoulders are relaxed, his head is down and his eyes are downcast. He should wait quietly without fidgeting. If his knees are not open wide enough for you to see his genitals from where you are sitting, kick or push them apart with your foot until you are satisfied with their spread.

Position Four

If Position Three is "at-ease" then Position Four is "attention." Position Four is a waiting/inspection position. It has some aspects of Two, the standing inspection position, and some aspects of Three, "at-ease."

What you do: Call "four" from a seated or standing position.

What he does: His butt snaps up off his heels and he assumes an upright kneeling position. The upward movement should be crisp and sharp, just as if he were snapping to "attention." His hands drop to his sides and rest palms-in toward his thighs. This should happen naturally as he rises. His head is down and his eyes are downcast as he awaits your pleasure.

Position Five

Position Five is designed to test the obedience and humility of the slave. It is the position for a kneeling inspection and never have I met a slave that could withstand its appeal.

What you do, part one: Call "five" from a comfortable stance.

What he does: He drops to his knees, sits on his heels and opens his feet and knees. Again, the drop should be more like sinking down and very graceful. As he sits on his heels, the motion should be controlled, not a plopping down. Then he bends over and touches his forehead to the floor. His hips are held high. Reaching back with both arms, he grasps a buttock in each hand and spreads his cheeks for your inspection.

What you do, part two: Circle him slowly, making it clear from your gait and stance that you *are* inspecting him. Place one finger on his buttock as you step around his feet. Nudge his feet farther apart with your foot. If he is responding to this well, try another verbal command. Tell him to "release his cheeks," pause a few seconds, and say slowly, "spread . . . ." How will you know if he likes this? Or anything else, for that matter? Does he have a hard-on? Does he have a glazed look around the eyes? Is he breathing heavily? Panting? Good!

Although I have made this into a "position" for training, this exact position is used by many dominants for many different reasons. In this context, I use it to impress his status as slave upon him and to make him proud to be one. Humbling, and exposing, himself to me should be natural since he is mine to do with as I wish. This position is also popular in mental bondage and slave training. Since it is a common, and very exciting, fantasy to be made to expose oneself to the unobstructed gaze of the dominant, if this is one of his fantasies, the word "five" should make him blanche with feigned distress.

Position Six

Position Six is a cute one I call "present nipples." Men's nipples are so shy, so sensitive, so demure compared to our full, luscious ones that I can't resist the temptation to coax them out of hiding and clamp things onto them!

What you do: Sit comfortably on your throne and say "six."

What he does: Position Six is similar to four in that he remains in the same upright kneeling position but in Position Six he crosses his arms behind the small of his back. As you can see, this thrusts his pecs out. His head is down and his eyes are downcast—since I am playing with his nipples, I want him to see what I am doing! Now make sure his shoulders are back. Don't his nipples look cute? Go ahead, give them a little tweak! Aren't they sensitive? Did he jump? Maybe even gasp in pain? What about his cock? Is it hard? Give it a gentle slap, quickly, before he realizes what you're going to do!

Position Seven

Position Seven is the position of confession. When he has been disobedient or has displeased me somehow, this is the position I have him assume while I speak to him about his infraction and tell him his punishment.

What you do: Sit or stand and assume the proper demeanor for his 'fessing up.

What he does: He is kneeling directly in front of you. His feet and knees are open and his buttocks are resting on his heels. His hands, curled into fists, rest knuckles down on either side of his knees. His shoulders are forward, as if he is ashamed of himself, his head is down and his eyes are downcast. His whole demeanor, the set of his shoulders, the way he hangs his head, should speak to you of his willingness to accept your verbal correction and corporal punishment, if you deem it necessary.

Position Eight

After confession comes forgiveness, and Position Eight is the position of forgiveness. He can beg your forgiveness either before or after his punishment or correction, whichever you prefer.

What you do, part one: Stand imperiously.

What he does: He is in the upright kneeling position (attention) to the right of your feet. His back is straight but his head is bowed and rests against your hip in an attitude of supplication. His arms are wrapped around your leg as if they, too, are pleading for your forgiveness. The occasional whimper or plea of "please, mistress, forgive me" is sweet music to your ears. He remains this way until you give him a sign he has been forgiven.

What you do, part two: Show him you forgive him by stroking his hair or patting his head, give him some little sign of endearment that shows him all is well and you have accepted him back into your good graces.

Position Nine

Position Nine is another waiting/inspection position and similar to the start position in the party game "Ruffs."

What you do: Command him to assume Position Nine.

What he does: He sinks gracefully to his knees then gets on all fours. His knees are as far open as his shoulders are wide. His hands are flat on the floor and the fingers are closed; the feet are bottoms up. His head is up and his eyes are looking straight ahead. His spine is straight and doesn't bend in the middle.

I like this position to keep him close to me in crowded places where, of course, he is allowed to move his head. In more private moments, I use this position to perform a different kind of inspection. Rather than inspect his "parts," I inspect him like one would inspect a possible mode of transportation. I step (gently!) on his fingers, I kick him lightly in the rump and thighs, I sit on shoulders, maybe even give a little bounce or two to test the shocks. I grab a tuft of his hair and use it to pull his head this way and that, testing him for compliance.

Position Ten

The final training position, Position Ten, is a neat little number that leaves him neatly tucked away at your feet or alternatively, tucked under your feet as an ottoman or footstool.

What you do: Sit there, say "ten." If you like, you can follow the verbal command with a hand signal: a finger pointing to the floor beside your feet might mean you want him neatly tucked up and out of the way; a pointing of the toe to the spot where you would like him, combined with the command "there" will give you a perfectly positioned footstool.

What he does: The position is the same for either command; what differs is where he assumes it. Either beside your feet or under them. He drops to his knees in that same graceful manner he has surely perfected by now. Again, he sits back on his heels. This time, when he bends forward his buttocks do not leave his heels. His hands are on either side of his knees, fingers closed. His head is between his hands, forehead on the floor. His elbows are neatly tucked in at his sides and his back is a slightly rounded, pleasing arc.

You can either walk around him and inspect him, correcting mistakes in his posture and commenting on his general appearance or you can just sit down and put your feet up.

Punishment Positions

Punishment positions are as numerous as the infractions that earn the punishments and as varied as the slaves that assume the positions. To get you started, I have laid out a set of positions, one for spanking (OTK), one for caning, and one for whipping. As you increase your repertoire and gain more exposure to D&S through reading and perhaps other couples, you can add any number of variations and entire new positions to this basic set.

Over-the-Knee (or OTK) Spanking

The classic position over your knee can be varied by sitting on a sofa rather than a chair. For the chair position, he will need to brace himself by putting his hands on the floor. I prefer the sofa. On the sofa, he can stretch out full length and concentrate on taking a harder, or longer, spanking rather than whether or not he's going to fall off your lap. Additionally, if the spanking is for punishment or correction rather than my pleasure, in the on-the-sofa variation, I can order him to clasp his hands behind the small of his back, thereby adding to his discomfort and his sense of helplessness.

Present

"Present" is any punishment position whereby he spreads his feet up to eighteen inches apart, bends at the waist and holds on to something: a desk, a chair, the arm of the sofa. Or sometimes, he holds on to thin air and just pretends there is something there. I use this position for caning, cropping, paddling, and whipping, or flogging. When you call for him to "present," he should immediately go to the piece of furniture you have indicated and assume the position over it. This position leaves his buttocks and upper back exposed for the attentions of the flogger or whip and presents a clear target for the caning, cropping, or paddling of the buttocks.

The Cross

This is my favorite position for him to assume to take a standing-up whipping or flogging. For this, you will need to tie his wrists to something: from the "Bondage" chapter, use simple wrist bondage combined with an over-the-door/doorknob restraint. The popular variation on the standing cross is to simply tie him, spread-eagled, to the bedposts or bed frame. As I mentioned in bondage, some people have deep fears about being tied spread-eagle to anything so make sure this is okay with him before you tie him up.

The variations are endless: put him on his back and hold his legs up by the ankles then paddle him (carefully!), or put him on all fours as in Position Nine, then straddle his head and clench it between your knees as you use the flogger or crop on him; discipline him with the whip or flogger while he is in Position Five. Those with simpler tastes might enjoy being tied, face-down, to the bed—a very comfortable position for him and hopefully, you will be able to flog him from three sides. Scout around for a used massage table or an examination table; most fold in half for easy storage and portability and make terrific D&S gear.

～ 12 ～

Role-Playing

Called "psychodrama" by many professionals and trendies, role-playing leads you to believe that each time you become the mistress you are playing a role. This is not always true. Sometimes couples are simply themselves during a scene where the main drama is the exchange of power, not the adopting of another persona and play-acting. I use role-playing to imply something outside the scope of a classic mistress/slave scenario.

While engaged in role-playing, you can become any one of a variety of people. Age-play fantasies are a classic theme where the dominant assumes the role of aunt, teacher, or other authority figure. British men seem to prefer school mistress and student fantasies. Another British favorite is that he has been sent to you, a correctional mistress, by his regular mistress for additional discipline. That usually means caning. Being a hostage of some sort is another popular scenario, as is being "run in" by a female officer of the law.

Role-playing doesn't involve discipline as a matter of course; in some fantasies, corporal punishment is inappropriate. In some cases, this is easy to figure out; in others, it is not. In a fantasy where he wants to be dressed as a woman and be "girlfriends" together, it isn't hard to figure out a beating is not in order here unless specifically asked for. As we discussed in "Cross-Dressing," this is what I call a total beauty session. The new "she" wants to be admired and convincingly treated like a girl.

Alternatively, a naughty boy caught dressing up in mommy's clothes might just want a beating dressed as a girl.

One of the hardest things for a budding domina to do is stay "in character" for an hour or longer. When I first started doing sessions, I quickly discovered that any break in the action made whatever happened next seem anticlimactic. So stopping the scene to ask him if he is ready to move on to the next phase of the fantasy is not advised. Smooth segues from one phase of the fantasy to the next should be planned. As the domina, it is up to you to regulate the progression of the action.

I have been asked to portray a young aunt, school mistresses, psychiatrists, a man, prison wardens, "lady" bosses, a secretary getting back at a boss who was sexually harassing her, a cop, a warden, a drill sergeant to a cross-dressed ex-marine and, separately, to a demolitions expert (both combined with verbal humiliation) and numerous more.

The "Action" Session

Once in a while a really unusual fantasy comes along. What makes it unusual is the scope of it, the topic itself, or any one of a number of things. My favorite psychodrama was the one I enacted with Max.

The scenario was that I was a cruel mistress and he was my newest slave. He was in the "city apartment" beginning his slave training. If his performance was unsatisfactory, he would be brought to my castle dungeon outside the city for the ultimate punishment.

I had received several hours' notice this session was going to happen so I had plenty of time to prepare. (There are those three P's again!) He had been very specific about his punishments. He asked that shaving be one. He also expressed an interest in being ridden like a pony and treated like a dog.

This is the rare fantasy a mistress dreams about. Plenty to work with and a touch of humor for good measure. I developed a plan. Always have one—a good one leaves room for spontaneity. I got a small plastic bag from the kitchen. Then I went into the bathroom and proceeded to trim my pubic hairs, careful to catch them in the baggie. I knew he would recognize them for what they were. After all, nothing looks like pubic hair except pubic hair.

He was naked, on his knees as I had instructed, when I made my entrance. I took my place of honor and instructed him how to address me, what positions I preferred him in, all the usual stuff. After receiving his homage, I whipped out the plastic bag and shook it under his nose. I demanded he tell me what was in the bag. His eyes opened wide as it dawned on him what it was. "Pubic hair, Mistress Claudia," his voice actually quivered. Impressed with my ingenuity, he was mine.

In a casual voice I told him the hair was a fellow slave's, I had overseen the shaving myself. I told him I had done this for no other reason than to show him I was serious about punishing him for his disobedience or poor performance. Well, I was supposed to be a cruel mistress, wasn't I?

Placing a chain choke collar around his neck, I told him he was now my dog. When I was growing up, my family always had a dog. At one time, we lived next door to a vet. So I know how dogs behave and how to treat them. So did he. But he didn't know I knew and I didn't know he knew. Again, I impressed him, this time with my intimate knowledge of doggie-dom.

He heeled nicely on his leash, sat, stayed, rolled over, begged, and barked to my satisfaction, but when I progressed to "fetch," he picked up the ball with his hand and stuffed it in his mouth. This is not allowed—dogs don't have hands! I hit him on the nose with a rolled up newspaper (something I would *never* do to a real dog!) and picked up the phone and ordered my dungeon staff to prepare the equipment to shave his body as punishment for his disobedience.

After that we moved on to pony rides. I love pony rides, and since there was no saddle, I had to ride bareback. I was sitting on his upper back with my legs wrapped around his middle and my ankles crossed in front of him. We weren't using a bridle because he was afraid for his dental work considering that the "bit" was actually a bar gag. In my left hand, I had a handful of his hair, which I used as reins to keep me on his back. In my right hand, I had my lovely riding crop. I was cropping him around the room, and to this day, I'm not sure what happened next. Maybe I gave him an extra vigorous blow, or clipped him with the tip of my crop in a delicate area, or maybe nothing happened at all. Maybe he just got a little frisky but in any case, he whinnied and reared up horse-style. And dumped me off his back into a heap on the floor! I landed on my back with a loud thump, my legs in the air still clinging to the mount that was no longer there, and an undominant yelp of surprise escaping from my lips.

My pony had a confused look on his face—should he humble himself before me and beg for mercy? Which end of me? Should he laugh? He was waiting for a clue from me. Figuring I couldn't retain my dignity and dominant mystique under such circumstances, I did the next best thing. I laughed. Now he was free to laugh with me. After all, it *was* funny. He assisted me to my feet in a gentlemanly manner, apologized in a suitably humble manner, and bore his punishment stoically.

Although we both laughed at my ignominious dismount, it gave me the opportunity to inflict the final punishment on him. Again, I picked up the phone and got my dungeon staff on the line. Their orders were to prepare for my arrival with the new slave within the hour. I hung up without signing off.

Taking his chin in my hand, I described to him in loving detail how it would feel to be shaven, and how it would itch when it grew in. I told him that the other slaves would know just by looking at him how much he had displeased me. I ordered him to dress and get in the car. To end the session, I left the room. It was a terrific session for both of us.

The Psychological Session

The role I played with Max was that of a cruel, sadistic mistress, whereas my normal mistress persona is one that treats her submissive as a pampered pet/body slave. And in Max's fantasy, there were many hands-on, physical things to do as well as the shaving fantasy/punishment. The role I played for Michael was that of a psychiatrist, and his fantasy was entirely psychological.

His fantasy was unusual in that I didn't really have to do anything but sit there, listen to him, and pump him for more information about his thoughts and feelings. I played his psychiatrist and he remained "himself." I was seated in my chair when he arrived. The door to the room was ajar a few inches, the "signal" that the doctor was in and ready to see him. He came to me, as his "psychiatrist," on a Tuesday to tell me that he had been arrested on Friday night for drunk driving and taken to jail. Incarcerated for the entire weekend, he was thrown into a cell with twelve to fourteen other men, all "real" criminals and felons. They begin to ridicule him and insult him, then it escalated to them encircling him and slapping him back and forth among them. They started to rip at his clothes, then he was knocked to the concrete floor of the cell and stripped by his humiliators.

As he related his fantasy degradations I asked him how he felt about being ridiculed and humiliated by these men, how he felt when they stripped him. Did he fight? At first, but there were too many of them. Did he have any bruises, black and blue marks? No, there were so many of them they didn't need to hit him, they simply overpowered him. And raped him. At first, one at a time while the others held him down, then one back and one front as he grew less and less resistant. By the time they were through with him, he was lying on the cell floor and they were standing around him in a circle, masturbating on him.

I asked why he had ceased to fight and how he felt being used by the men. He stopped fighting because it was useless, he protested, there were too many of them and he was afraid he would get hurt. Didn't he cry out? And what about the guards? He did but they didn't hear or didn't come, he didn't know and then his mouth was full. At first he was deeply degraded and shamed by their use of him, but by the end he had grown compliant. His compliance and its underlying consent shamed him and he needed to "talk" to someone about his experience in the jail. Many of the best humiliation fantasies center around coercion and ultimate consent.

As his "psychiatrist," I did little more than sit there and ask what I thought would be questions he would like to answer. He wanted to verbalize to someone his violent dream of rape and degradation to make it more real to himself. Obviously, it was much safer to see a "psychiatrist" and relate his "terrible" experience than it was to go out and *have* the terrible experience. This, I felt, was a balanced way of living out his fantasy in a harmless, secure surrounding with an understanding role-player. But as you can see, this session was very different from the one with Max.

The Character Session

Sometimes the role-playing fantasy takes the shape of a specific and known character, a public person, real or fictional, a television character, whomever, but let's say someone you can "research" to some extent. One truly popular character that mistresses love to play and slaves loved to be captured by is the inimitable Mrs. Emma Peel, of *The Avengers*, immortalized by the equally inimitable and enormously talented Diana Rigg.

Many of you, like me, may have been a Mrs. Peel fan when the show was in its prime. Her intelligence, courage, spunk, sense of humor, to say nothing of that marvelous '60s wardrobe, her fantastic job as counteragent/spy lady and the neat cars she got to ride around in, made her my heroine and the stuff of many a man's fantasy. This is a classic version of the captor/hostage scenario with a surreal twist. And very easy for you to dress for and enact. A black lycra and cotton catsuit, a body suit and leotards or very tight stretch pants, any leather at all: pants, skirt, vest, or motorcycle jacket and boots with a heel, and you're basically dressed as Mrs. Peel. A big belt slung around your hips would help complete the look or a leather cap if you're into leather would be a nice accessory.

One man who I saw several times had an Emma Peel fantasy and since playing Mrs. Peel was my favorite role, this was a match made in D&S heaven. One of our pet openers was one that required each of us to do some separate preparations. I did what I usually did, dressed, did my makeup and hair, and took out the equipment I wanted to use for this scene: a straight, low-backed chair, handcuffs and ankle shackles, two butter knives, a straight razor, and a large hunting knife. He was busy looking through his clothes to find old ones to wear (particularly a T-shirt, underwear, and a cloth belt) and packing a bag of replacements.

He would call from the corner pay phone and I would come down and kidnap him, grabbing him by the arm and holding a pointy finger into his ribs like a gun. Once in my apartment, I would cuff him hand and foot to the chair. Holding his head up at the chin with the point of the knife, I would tell him to save himself a lot of trouble. He would quiver and moan and protest that he didn't know anything, please, let him go, please. Then I'd step behind him and pull his head back by the hair; holding the knife to his throat (blade away from his neck!) I'd tell him I had ways to make him talk. Next, I would blindfold him. Taking the two butter knives, I would hold them next to his ear and rub them against each other in a "sharpening" motion which made a wonderful metallic hiss. Each hiss sent him into spasms of delicious fear at the cruelty and beauty of his captor.

After giving him one more opportunity to talk, I would use the hunting knife and the straight razor to relieve him of his old clothes, one little piece at a time. Sometimes I would cut the T-shirt off starting at the neck, straight down to his cloth belt. Other times, I would pull out and cut off a circular patch to expose each nipple, leaving the rest of the shirt intact until that, too, fell under "my knife." We had agreed to leave his pants intact, so after cutting his cloth belt open, I would remove his pants myself, usually leaving them just below his knees to add to the feeling of being restrained. Then I would slowly (and carefully!) cut away his underwear. All of this was done in front of a floor to ceiling mirror in a darkened room with black leather furniture, and it was very, very sexy and empowering.

"Mr. Peel" and I had many fun nights together as Mrs. Peel and her captive. To further enhance our scenarios, he brought me a set of long and short samurai swords, a skinning knife, another hunting knife, and a very pretty gravity knife. We would fence in my living room, moving the furniture up against the walls to give us more floor space. I'd watch karate movies and try the moves on him. With his full cooperation, I was able to throw him around the room, knock him to his knees, and win at fantasy wrestling. This was terrific fun for me. As I weigh only 105 pounds, most men can pick me up and twirl me like a baton without breaking a sweat! And here I was, tossing him around the room like a rag doll! Then, having worked up a tremendous appetite from all this physical activity, we'd don our street clothes and go out for a bite.

Fortunately, there is lots of Mrs. Peel stuff around if you want to do some fun homework. Several cable stations rerun *The Avengers* and several books covering the show and/or Mrs. Peel may still be available. Or maybe you prefer to be Bonnie Parker. Or the Empress Josephine. Or the

Red Queen. Think of the fun you can have commanding "off with his head," leaving him to wonder which one you are talking about!

But in case you haven't been fortunate enough to be presented with a role you think you can pull off, discuss this with your mate right away. This would be in the negotiating period right before you give the signal to let the games begin. Often small adaptations, or omissions, can solve the problem.

A personal quirk of mine is feeling bad about hitting a woman. This extends to a man dressed as a woman. Yet this is a common fantasy combination. And knowing they want to be hit doesn't help. So I don't give "women" beatings anymore. But I will beat him before I dress him up, or after she's changed back into a "man," and tie it in that way. He gets his due and I don't do anything that makes me uncomfortable.

The Bitch Session

"Cupcake" is a good-looking, trim, clean-smelling man in his mid-thirties. He was my foot slave for many years. I gave him the mercy word "cupcake" because it was unlikely we'd ever be talking about cupcakes in a session. I began calling him Cupcake to tease him. When I first met him, he was only interested in foot worship. However, there are things I like to do too, so we negotiated beforehand what his limit was that day. And I would take him to that limit. If he took it well, I would try to take him a little further.

He liked his first beating so much that soon he was begging me to give him another (my pleasure, slave!). And then to hit him a little harder. Or to use the riding crop, not the suede cat. We progressed to bondage at my suggestion, blindfolding at his. One role-play game I played with him was called "Shoe Store."

He was the hapless salesman, dressed in a leather G-string I had gotten him. I was the bitch/goddess customer, arrogant, demanding, hard to please. I went so far as to step out in the hall and ring my own bell. He opened the door for me, took my coat and escorted me to my chair, all in a very subservient manner.

You already know I have an irrational shoe fetish myself, so I naturally have all my precious darlings in separate plastic boxes, lined with tissue paper, so they don't get scuffed or dusty. I have several pairs that have never been worn in the street. I carry them to where I am going and change inside. Others have never been worn outside of my apartment. There were over a dozen pairs of shoes laid out for me to try on and I tried on every single pair of them, some more than once. He was to slavishly admire me as I paraded around the room and posed in the mirror wearing the shoes. He was to slip each shoe on and off my foot, never letting my foot touch the floor. We played this game for almost two hours. In spite of this lovely game I dreamed up, he was so afraid I wasn't going to give him his beating that he requested one.

Although "Shoe Store" is a mild game, the point of this is he trusted me enough to respect his limits to allow me to test them. Remember, when I first began seeing him, he was only interested in straight, so to speak, foot worship. His range of interests expanded over the five years I saw him, making our time together that much more interesting and satisfying for both of us. This is a perfect progression in the role of Mistress/Slave. It means you, the domina, have played your role very well. I got a great deal of personal satisfaction out of Cupcake's progress.

Age-Play Scenarios

A very popular age-play scenario is that of the student being corrected by the schoolmistress. In America, men into this fantasy favor the paddle as the means of discipline. British and European men favor the cane for punishment. In the real world where the boys were exposed to this type of punishment, certain "rituals" took place prior to the actual beating. In America, the young man was told to leave the class and wait out in the hall. Then the teacher followed with her paddle (each desk seems to have come with its own). After ascertaining that the young man knew what he was being punished for, the mistress would rub the paddle on his bottom three times before giving him three hard whacks. The second infraction earned five hard whacks. Then they would simply return to the classroom, to the snickers of those left inside.

In Britain, caning was the most popular form of punishment used at boys schools. I have no information as to whether or not women were caned, too. The major difference in the two scenarios is that in the British variation, the young man was called after school to receive his punishment and could go home afterward instead of face his classmates right away. (Unless they were waiting for him to "see" how he did!)

Infantilism

It will come as no surprise that infantilism is role-play involving infantlike behavior such as wearing and soiling a diaper, nursing, sucking a bottle or pacifier, and wanting to be burped or rocked to sleep. The scientific term for infantilism is "autonepiophilia," which is enough of a reason to call it something else. But no matter what you call it, it is probably the least understood and most belittled of all role-play/age-play fantasies. Because of their penchant for dressing and acting like babies, infantilists (who only age-play with other adults) are often mistaken for pedophiles. The infantilist usually is not a pedophile and is often protective of children, but, the misunderstanding of his motives and the fantasies of such helplessness as that of an infant make even some D&Sers uncomfortable.

A number of professional dominants have special nursery equipment built to scale for their big babies. Authenticity is a main concern and an erotic requirement. Toys and clothes must fit the age of the infant as should the child's behavior. My friend Amanda sees a man we call "Baby Leo" for four- and five-hour sessions. During that time she changes his diaper, burps him, puts him "down for a nap," feeds him, and plays baby games with him. Baby Leo goes to the local fetish parties in his baby gear, walks around sprinkling baby powder everywhere, then sits down right in the middle of things and cries "WAAAHHH!" Amanda assures me that "babies" are very demanding.

Juvenility

In this age-play fantasy, he dreams he is a young boy again, not an infant, but a boy of anywhere from five on up to twelve or thirteen. As in infantilism, authenticity is a main ingredient in style of dress, speech, and manner for the "young" man and his role-player in juvenility. Often, some mode of humiliation is incorporated into the fantasy. It could be relating to him embarrassing tales of his "younger" days. One client liked to be told that I had taught him how to hold his willie and aim his stream into the toilet bowl. Another wanted to be brought into the ladies' room to relive his bladder, just like his mother had done (and probably many other mothers just like her!). Many who have this type of fantasy long for the carefree days of childhood and feel relaxed for days after a juvenility session.

Adolescence

Again in the age-play fantasy, adolescence is the next age up from juvenility. These men fantasize that they are teenagers once more, ranging in age from thirteen to eighteen. This is the most common fantasy age group as many boys either first become interested in girls at this age, had their first sexual experience at this age, or had discipline fantasies. Interestingly, several men I spoke to who indulged in this fantasy said that their first experience was with an older woman, either an aunt or cousin, a friend's mother or a neighbor, and they went forward from there. These fantasies encompass all sorts of interests since he is old enough in this fantasy to have had some life experience and make a choice as to his favorite things or things he would like to experiment with. If you have ever had fantasies about being with a sweet, fresh young man, you and this dreamer-of-younger days were made for each other!

Doggie Obedience School

In the chapter on Humiliation, we spoke about objectification fantasies where the submissive acts the part of the mistress's pet. Alternatively, some players consider becoming your "pet" a role to be played rather than an object to become, since pets, like a dog or a cat, exhibit distinct personalities. One of the most popular requests from men who like to indulge in this kind of role-playing, especially beginners, is to be treated like your dog, in the literal sense. This is a very simple game to play and your don't need much, or expensive, equipment to play it.

All you really need to start is a leash and a collar and you may already have the collar if you have chosen that to be the symbol of his slavery. If the slave collar you have chosen is a leather collar, perhaps you may want to pick out a chain choke collar for him (be careful with it!) if being your dog is his fantasy, or yours. If you have ever had a dog, this role will be easy for you to assume. Think back and remember what your dog used to do on his own and also how you played with him and disciplined him. (Of course, you never hit a real dog with a rolled-up newspaper. I reserve that particular punishment for human dogs.) If he has ever had a dog, it will be easy for him to step into the role also. Below are suggestions for people who have never had a dog and need a little coaching in the ways of our four-legged friends. In the "Party Games" chapter, you have read how to play the game "Ruffs." This is an excellent dog training manual.

Since he is now your dog, the standard positions for a slave to assume do not apply here. Every time he moves away from your chair, he should be on all fours just like a dog. If you want him to lie down, proper dog positions include stretched out full length with his head between his "paws," and on his side with his front and back legs close to each other. Proper sitting positions include sitting on his rump with both legs to one side, his forelegs out in front of him to support himself and the classic sitting dog position—sitting squarely on his rump with his back legs out to each side and his front legs between them, again to support himself. This is the more difficult of the two positions since it is harder for him to stay in this position for any length of time.

Now that he knows how to sit and lie down like a dog, what else do dogs do? Well, they pant to cool themselves off. This is pretty easy as well as self-explanatory. But if he doesn't know how to do it, teach him. Open your mouth and extend your tongue so it rests on your lower lip. It should project out over your lip just about a half an inch. Then pant. Every once in a while, draw your tongue back into your mouth and swallow.

Dogs also eat their food and drink out of bowls on the floor. Get a little placemat and make that his eating area. I have regular dog bowls for my slave, one for his water and one for his food. I don't actually feed him dog food, I feed him chili because it looks like dog food and unlike real dog food, I know he will eat it. (It helps that I make great chili.) Make sure he laps up his water doggie style, with his tongue, and eats his food the same way. As a dog treat, I get a piece of cake or a corn/bran muffin and shape it into dog bone shapes with a knife. I use these "treats" to reward him for learning a new trick or obeying a command, just as I did with my real dogs.

Then there are a whole variety of commands you can give him, like sit, stay, fetch, beg, roll over, play dead, speak, and sing. You can leash train him by teaching him to heel, stop when you stop, and keep the same pace as you. You can also train him to stay when you walk away from him and come when you call him. For particularly bright dogs, you can teach him how to walk himself. This entails carrying the end of his leash in his mouth and still keeping step with you. When you say "speak" he should bark in a realistic manner, more like a "ruff, ruff" than a bowwow. Singing, in doggie-dom, is when the dog throws back his head and howls wolf-style, like baying at the moon.

You could also consider laying out newspaper for him as if you were housebreaking a puppy. It doesn't matter whether or not he actually uses the paper, but it presents a realistic visual image for him and impresses his status as your dog on him. For each successfully completed command, you can reward him with a "dog bone" or a scratching behind his ears (a big favorite with real dogs), or a rubbing on his belly (a big favorite with human and real dogs). The customary disobediences are failing to carry out a command, pulling on his leash, not bringing the ball back to you, barking for no reason, and missing the newspaper when he piddles!

Role-playing is territory just waiting to be explored—by you! You can be anyone you can dream up, real or imaginary, then dress for the part and play "pretend" till your heart's content. The more exotic the fantasy, the more fun you can have with it. Some favorite fantasy scenarios include "Hijacker or Terrorist/Steward/ess," "GI Joe/Enemy," "Warden/Prisoner," and "Schoolmistress/Student." Favorite role-playing combinations include elder sister/younger brother, nurse or doctor/patient, wicked stepmother/stepson, aunt/nephew, cop/perpetrator, schoolmistress/student, warden or prisoner guard/inmate, and a vast variety of other combinations. Personally, when I'm playing the dominant I like to be Cleopatra, Bathsheba, the Tsaress (as in Catherine the Great), Vera the Slave Trainer, Lady Executive, Bitch Goddess, a queen, princess, cop, and on and on depending on what day it is.

~ 13 ~

Sensation

In its own sexy little way, sensation in D&S play is (al)most addic-
tive. An Englishman I know once called himself a "sensation slut"
because he liked all types of pain rather than just those caused by
corporal punishment. Nipple clamps, ice, waxing, and anal play all provide exquisite sensations for the submissive outside the discipline context. Imaginative lot that we are, D&Sers regularly experiment with
sensation and intense stimulation. You could say that sensation is a further exploration into the eroticism of discomfort.

A method called "conditioning" is employed by the dominant to
train the submissive to respond to pain stimuli the same as he would to
pleasure. Scientifically put, stimulus association (what D&Sers call "conditioning") occurs when two stimuli repeatedly occur together and
become associated with each other. Anyone can be conditioned to
respond erotically to noneortic stimuli with a little time and patience.
An example of conditioning is in the "Discipline" chapter.

One of my slaves furnishes a nice example of conditioning. At first,
he came to me only for light bondage: his own exercise in helplessness.
I insisted on giving him a beating because I like to give them. I assured
him it would be a beginner's beating, more like a hard caress than a
whipping, and if he didn't like it, he could say his safe word and I
would stop immediately. He didn't say his safe word.

Next, I tried nipple clamps on him. I would put them on after his
dog collar and before his cock rings. I called it "dressing him in chains."

He liked it. Then, I progressed to hot wax. After that I was able to coax him into some light genital bondage and then a light genital whipping. Over our time together, I have come to notice a few things about him. As I just said, originally he was just a light bondage enthusiast. If the bondage scene was good, he had quite an erection. For the beating, it was considerably less strong. And then I began to notice that even if he was in his favorite kind of bondage, when I was not whipping his genitals his erection flagged a bit.

That is just a one example of how you can condition your partner to accept some pain, and then more pain with or without beating him.

Pain

I think pain, in general, is a misunderstood concept. Pain itself is neither good nor bad, it is just another sensation. A good beating *feels* good. And most people who are into pain as a pleasure source do not want to be beaten to within an inch of their lives. These people are very rare and usually still need the buildup in order to take their full dosage of pain.

Additionally, there are many levels of pain to be experienced. The first and gentlest level could be called a "sensuous massage". This level of "pain" is for those who only want the sensation of being whipped. It usually begins with soft caresses, touching, and teasing; some tops use a "bunny cloth" of fur or a wool mitt, feathers, or long, light strokes of their fingernails to enhance the sensation. Then it is followed up with a light whipping using a deerskin flogger. For some, the "pain" stops here; for others, this is the initial or warm-up stage. For those who wish to continue to explore pain and take it to the next level, as sexual arousal occurs, heavier, harder strokes and more severe instruments can be used by the top.

Another warm-up technique for more experienced or masochistic players uses a mixture of pleasure and pain that also allows a gradual buildup but begins at a higher pain level. Some tops throw one hard stroke in amongst the soft or more moderate ones, for example, producing a sharper "ouch" response that at first hurts then hurts so good. This is a little tricky because the bottom has to be feeling sexual *before* you begin whereas in the first method, the "beating" itself makes the bottom feel sexual.

Then there is the love/hate pain. Many of you will probably experience the first two types but this one is in the realm of The Perverati. Personally, this would be the type of pain masochists associate with a pleasurable caning, but it can happen with a whip, paddle, crop, anything. The pain of the stroke is an easily endured pain, like a cane when it lands. Then the fun begins. The pain of the stroke subsides and a new pain sets in. This is a feeling of great warmth, or even hotness, that ripples or radiates away from where the blow was landed.

When the cane lands, there is a hot slash of pain where it hits. That is the initial pain, the pain that is endurable. But even that pain raises the slave's upper body up off the bench or sofa arm. Then the second wave of pain hits. An electric jolt radiates out from that area. One wave heads for the genitals and the other wave rockets up the spine, setting each vertebrae ablaze en route to the brain. The wave hits the brain stem and explodes throughout the head in a white hot brilliant starburst of agony followed by intensely erotic feelings. Or an orgasm. A rhythm is created between the top and bottom and the cane and the slave dances in exquisite pain to the tune I play on his body. Like scotch, this kind of pain is an acquired taste and it will probably be some time before the two of you reach this level.

Punitive pain, the final level of pain is the most extreme, not necessarily because of the pain level itself but because this type of pain is not erotic, nor is it meant to be. Punitive pain is pain as punishment and I am all for it in the D&S context. Within the D&S community, however, there is some small debate over the "validity" of punitive pain; exponents state that punitive pain is a destructive element. But what if you are training him to obedience and he disobeys? If his preference is for pain, why shouldn't the pain be punitive, be his punishment? Arguments against say that punitive pain can erode the hard earned trust of a D&S relationship and may lead to abuse. Those against punitive pain say that just ignoring the slave is punishment enough.

I don't see it. We are not talking about anyone of us living a constant D&S lifestyle, we are talking about a few hours of negotiated playtime! Many bottoms really like being punished for misbehaving and understand the difference between punishment and abuse. Many of these misbehave so they can be punished when they feel the mistress is taking too long. I call these "frisky" slaves. Told we were going to play "fetch," the slave would charge up to me and snatch the ball from my hand with his mouth before I could toss it! He loved to earn beatings for being frisky. Why deny these spirited souls their pleasure?

Nipple Clamps, Clips, and Clothespins

Because of their shy and retiring nature, many women overlook men's nipples as an erogenous zone. I find their nipples to be extremely sensitive and responsive. Pinch them gently at first, squeezing your fingers together as if they were going to meet in the middle. Pulling his nipples while you are pinching them is excitingly painful, too. But I don't recommend twisting them; most people don't enjoy it. His nipples can be especially usefully in their capacity to train him to associate pain with pleasure.

Basically, what a nipple clamp does is cut off the circulation of blood to his nipple. The first sensation is pain when the clamp is applied to it. Secondly, they may develop almost a numb ache after the initial pain subsides. After that, he will become more accustomed to them and they will only hurt him when you pull on them or attach weights.

But there is a hidden agenda. Remember the numb ache? The numb ache was his circulation being cut off. When you release the clamp, his blood will rush into his nipple. The flow of blood rushing back into that part of his body will cause him infinitely more pain than the first application of the clamps. His nipples will remain very sensitive for several minutes after the clamps have been removed.

Conduct a little experiment on your partner's nipples. Pinching and pulling them the way I described above, beginning gently, try it on him and observe his reaction. Some men, like women, have extremely sensitive nipples and can't take any pain in this area at all. If his reaction seems sincere, nipple clamps are not for you. But you can always use your fingers, or threaten him with them if you want, or need, to. If his reaction is good, then you have a whole new area to play with. And maybe even some new toys to buy.

Often I have heard people recommend wooden clothespins as nipple clamps. I have done so myself, right in this book. However, wooden clothespins are merciless unless they are older, loosened up ones. The plastic kind that look like kids toys in pastel colors are better for the beginner. I feel it is better to invest in a pair of regular nipple clamps if he passes the fingertip test. Two of the three kinds recommended below are adjustable and one can be adjusted easily with a pair of pliers.

Of the many different kinds, my favorite are the Japanese clover clamps. I see a gracefulness in the mechanism that makes them pleasing to my eye. I like the way the chain connects them, either up to the ring in his collar or just draped against his chest. Sometimes, I have him hold the chain in his mouth so that he pulls on his own nipples. This kind can be adjusted with pliers if the grip is too tight.

The next kind I favor are tonglike. With a chain attaching them, these clamps look like tweezers with a ring that slides down to make them tighter. And hold them that way. These are good for beginners because they are not too cruel and can be bent easily with just your fingers to adjust the bite. The ends of these are also covered with black or red insulation or plastic to protect his tender flesh.

The third kind of nipple clamp is the clip type, or alligator clamp. For the beginner I would recommend the ones with the screws to adjust the tension in the tip and with the protective plastic insulation which is usually red or black plastic. Nipple clamps should always be removed by unscrewing and/or unclipping them, not by pulling.

A few things to keep an eye out for when nipple playing: check the skin under the clip or clamp or pin to make sure it isn't being cut or irritated. Clamps, clips or pins should not be left on overly long, fifteen to twenty minutes at most depending on where, but remember, everyone is different, so watch his body language and listen to him.

Hot Wax

A personal favorite of mine, hot wax is play-painful but not really painful, if you do the waxing correctly. The bottom likes waxing because of the erotic unpredictability of where the wax will fall and the heat of it mixing with other sensations. For the dominant it is a power trip because she can apply the wax anyplace that strikes her fancy then remove it by whipping it off him or by carefully and slowly scraping the hardened wax off him with the blunt side of a knife. For quick removal, often with the wax coming off in one piece like a mold of that body part, slather him in moisturizer before coating him in wax.

Never use plastic coated candles because the wax gets very hot and can actually burn him. Dyed candles burn hotter and raise the temperature of the wax, making them unsatisfactory for use. Some hot-waxers prefer beeswax candles just because they get so very hot. I would not advise this for a beginner; remember you have to build him up to it slowly so you don't scare him off. I tried tapers and votive candles, but it was a little difficult to get the wax to land exactly where I wanted it. Just to be safe, I would experiment on myself to determine the distance from the body and the amount of time needed for the wax to cool off or to be a comfortable temperature before using it on him.

I prefer the white, undyed, unscented candles that come in the jelly-jar-size glasses. Many supermarkets sell them for under a dollar. With these candles, I found I had the most control over where the wax went (because I could pour it out of the glass) and how much of it came out. Also, since the melted wax is held in the glass, I was able to build up a reservoir of wax to torture him with. This method ensures that the wax will be medium hot, hot enough to give him the sensation but not too hot to burn him.

I light the candles when he arrives and let the wax melt and build up in the glass. When there is enough in the glass, about an inch, you will have enough to use on him effectively. By lighting many candles, you will have a ready supply of wax. Blow the candle out and wait for the wax to cool some. Less time if you want the wax hotter and more time if you want it cooler. The top layer of the wax will be cooler than the wax on the bottom. So don't be too hasty. Dip a pinkie all the way down to test for temperature. And remember that different parts of the body react to heat differently, so what's pleasurable on his buttocks may be too hot for his nipples or his cock.

Position him however you like, depending on where you want the wax to go. If you want it to run down his back, have him kneeling in front of you, leaning forward. If you want it to collect in a pool, or want to make a "design" with the drippings, have him lie down. Now that he is in position, hold the candle about twelve to eighteen inches over him.

If you hold it any closer, the wax will be very hot, too hot, and may turn him off to further encounters of this nature.

Aim for the good spots—his nipples and upper chest and, when you turn him over, his buttocks. As time goes on, he may even enjoy it dripped on his genitals.

A couple of pointers on hot waxing. Let it dry completely before you remove it. Dried wax is especially difficult to get out of hair so if your partner is a hairy guy you should take this into consideration. Slathering him with moisturizer before waxing him will ease the removal of that waxy buildup! Also, a cloth wet with cold water placed on the wax can help it to harden and aid you in removing any recalcitrant pieces of it you haven't been able to pull off with your fingers. If you pull the wax off quickly, you are likely to remove some of his body hair at the same time. Some people like this tiny torture. (It is just like having your legs waxed).

If his butt isn't hairy, I find that many enjoy having the wax whipped off their butts, just as it dries, with a moderate flogger. You hit just hard enough for the wax to be taken off and then you can continue until all of it is gone. And, if you happen to spill some on the carpet, place a paper towel over the waxy area and apply a medium iron to the paper towel. The wax will melt onto the towel and off of the rug.

Fire

I once saw on a special topics calendar at an S&M society an open discussion called "Playing on Submissives' Basic Fear of Fire and Needles." It was such a ridiculous, self-important title that I had to laugh. Submissive or not, if someone set your hair on fire, wouldn't you be a little fearful, maybe even a little upset? And needles? Well, I don't know about you but when I go to the dentist I have to be so knocked out on the nitrous oxide (sweet air or laughing gas) that I don't see the novocaine needle coming. Because if I do . . . I'm out in the street in a flash, with the little napkin and chain still hanging around my neck! It makes me wonder who these people are and if they are the same ones who are against punitive pain.

Since ancient times fire has been a source of wonder, fear, awe, and comfort. Fire itself is pure and metaphysical and, like time, it is an

implacable predator. As friend, fire is a source of light and warmth sym-
bolizing safety and security; as foe, fire becomes a threat to life. Concerned with nothing but its own lust and life, fire indiscriminately
consumes everything in its path. D&Sers are as fascinated with fire as
were the ancients, and use its magic and mystery to add to their scenes.

In its showiest form, some D&S dance teams have used fire as part
of overtly sexual performance art. This requires some training in the
proper use of green alcohol which is what burns rather than the skin or
other surface it is on. It is available in magic shops, most of which offer
a course in its use; some require the course before selling the products.

No, I don't expect many of you to run out and learn how to breathe
fire to impress your mate but there are a couple of fun, safe games with
fire that I guarantee will get his motor running.

You need a hairy mate for this or else a mate with a generous patch
of hair either on his chest or his pubis. Use a long fireplace match. If
he is blindfolded, strike it close enough to his face that he can smell the
sulfur. After the initial blaze or flare of the match has died down and it
is just a small steady flame, pass it back and forth over his chest hairs
or groin hairs. They sizzle up really fast but don't burn to the skin and
have a terrible smell, making it seem much worse than it really is. If he
tends to flop around like a landed fish during these playtimes, I would
tie him down before attempting this.

A client I saw had a twist on the scene. First he asked if I gave a
hard beating, then he was careful to inquire if I smoked. "Really smoke,
not fake it," he said. After being assured that I did both, the session was
set. He had pantyhose on when I arrived. Except for pulling them down
over his buttocks for the beating, he wore them the entire time. I was
dressed in a very tailored coatdress and black hose and pumps. We
began with a beating, skipping the sensitizing at his request. I started
with a moderate whip and quickly progressed to my riding crop.

After his backside was nicely crisscrossed with the thicker marks of
the crop, I switched to the cane. It hurts more, and also leaves marks
but thinner ones. A nice contrast to the crop marks, I thought. I beat
him very thoroughly with the cane before finishing it off with a few
strokes from my latex cord whip. He was limp on the bed, breathing
heavily, his bottom a mass of red marks left by the different implements.

Leaving the bedside, I sat in a chair and lit up, pretending to relax after having given such a strenuous beating. I puffed on my cigarette, making tons of smoke, steaming it up. When it was good and hot, I rolled the lighted tip into a point on the side of the ashtray. I ordered him to turn face up, and position himself spread-eagle on the bed. Then I dragged the lit end down the inside of his panty-hosed thigh several times, putting many runs in the hose and singeing a fair amount of his hair. And then I did it harder, brushing the light against his skin as I went.

For the grand finale, I ground out my cigarette on his inner thigh, right opposite the burn he had given himself. I was proud of myself, I wasn't sure I had it in me!

Ice

A little cube of ice, so small, so innocent, here now, gone so soon, can be an instrument of torture or a delicious respite for your submissive. Let's talk about the respite first.

After a paddling or spanking or any other corporal punishment that leaves the bottom's bottom hot and red all over, an ice cube trailed gently across his hot, red skin will be a nice cooling touch that will bring the temperature of his skin down slightly. After he adjusts to the initial shock of cold, he will thank you for this. Then you can continue with the ice cube or resume with the paddle, holding the ice cube in reserve for next time. Or feed it to him if he is thirsty.

Ice is also used in a waxing technique called "Fire and Ice" that is very visual and sexy but is pretty safe. Hot wax is poured on the submissive followed by a rubdown with ice to harden the wax faster. The contrast of the hot wet wax and the cold wet ice are exciting sensations; a good dominant will vary the amounts of each to keep up her reputation for being unpredictable.

The ice cube as an instrument of torture is discussed in the next subchapter.

Anal Play

Taboos about one's anus are ingrained in us from earliest childhood. The most pervasive negative attitudes are tied to the "uncleanliness" of the area and, for men, anal pleasure is closely associated with homosexual behavior. Because of this many adults, men and women, are alienated from their anuses and the erotic pleasures to be had there. Hidden between the folds of the buttocks, what the Marquis de Sade lovingly described as the "rosebud" opening is, for most people, anything but.

The personality of the anal taboo is a complex one. On one level it is taken for granted that the anal area is off-limits. The validity of the taboo is never questioned, like the taboo against eating the meat of dogs or cats. On a second level, since everyone is capable of receiving pleasure from anal play, negative messages from the mind often contradict the pleasurable feelings received from below. Additionally, in some religious societies the anal taboo is seen as coming directly from God. These religions insist that an inherent conflict always and forever exists between the body and the spirit and that one must be subjugated for the fulfillment of the other. And to that I say: Phooey! That kind of thinking foments internal conflict, increases feelings of guilt about otherwise delicious pleasures, and does nothing more than reinforce religious doctrine. I don't want these people in *my* bedroom, thank you.

Be that as it may, you are exploring your sexuality, enhancing and expanding it with every page you read. Because the anus has smells and textures unique to itself, it make take a while to develop a taste for play in this area. However, for a dominant woman, anal play can be a very exciting power trip; for a submissive, it is an extremely erotic act of submission. For some, anal relaxation and pleasure cannot be attained without a fantasy of being sexually overpowered: taken by force or swept away, perhaps tied up and then sodomized. These fantasies are not unusual in the D&S context. But, top or bottom, consenting to the nonconsensual or begging for the pleasure, the anus is a very delicate area, and certain precautions should be taken.

Since most people's distaste for their anus stems from feelings of uncleanliness, make sure the area is clean. This is accomplished with regular and careful washing. A good submissive will spend some time preparing for the session. This will usually include some sort of bathing, a full shower or bath or what I call a "birdbath": a full body wash with a cloth but under the bathtub faucet instead of in a full tub or shower. Make a bath or shower part of his "ritual of preparation" before playtime; then perform an "inspection" as described in "Positions" as part of your opening ritual if anal play is to be included. If penetration is part of the fantasy, you may want to give him, or instruct him to give himself, an enema. You can use the quart bag and/or Bardex types and administer the enema to him yourself as described in "Water Sports" as part of a power exchange or humiliation scene. Or you could direct him to give himself a Fleet from the drugstore without you. It is less personal and hands-on, but it will accomplish the same thing. It depends on the effect you want to have.

Speaking to the dominant, I would recommend that you use latex gloves, especially if you have a cut or scratch on your hand. Since he is your regular partner, transmission of sexually transmitted diseases (STDs) is not an issue here, but until you become used to playing in this area, you might be more mentally comfortable with the gloves. Everything that is to come in contact with or is to be put inside of the anus should be clean and very well lubricated. Latex gloves and condoms must be used with a water soluble, oil-free lubricant in order to preserve the integrity of the latex. Adult shops sell Astro-glide which I think is a wonderful vaginal or anal lubricant to use with latex protection; if all else fails, any local drugstore will sell old reliable, KY Jelly, which is a perfectly acceptable product for anal play. Avoid anything that contains a numbing agent—it will mask pain and tastes terrible if it gets on anywhere else.

There are several positions that the submissive can assume for anal play for maximum comfort and easy of entry, if that is your end goal: on his left side, his knees partially drawn up to his chest; or, on his belly with pillows under his hips elevating them to spread his cheeks; on his knees, his head and shoulders on the bed or floor (the kneeling inspection position); or on his back with his knees partially drawn up to his chest. I find this last position to be the least comfortable of the four unless the sphincter muscle has been relaxed and loosened beforehand.

Now we know he is clean inside and out and your hands are covered and lubricated. You may want to begin with him in the kneeling inspection position and just look at him for a minute. Make him aware that you are staring at his puckered brown opening and it, like the rest of him, is yours to do with as you please. If he likes this type of humiliation, he will be whimpering and panting by now. For an added touch, have him reach back, spread his cheeks and hold them open for you. Now, swipe a little lubrication on his anus in a wide paintbrush stroke, a whisper of a caress. Touch him gently because his anus will tense in fear of anticipated pain.

Before doing anything else, stroke his anus gently for a minute or two to allow him to adjust to "something" being there. This may be the first time he is trying anal play so make it a good experience for him. Caress him until you feel him relax. Now, try inserting one well lubricated finger into his anus. This is the most sensitive part of his anal anatomy and entry should be done slowly and gently. If his muscles are still too tight, you can just keep your finger there until he relaxes or you can coach him into compliance. Two things happen when something is inserted into the anus: the feeling of having to move one's bowels and the tensing of a muscle called the puborectal sling, which makes insertion more difficult. This is the muscle that is about 75 percent responsible for continence and, well, gas control. There are a couple of things he can do to help you in. First, he can bear down as if he is having a bowel movement; this will slacken the muscles some. If he is very focused, you could direct him to take ten deep breaths and concentrate on pushing down and out as he exhales. As he exhales, his anal muscle will relax and your finger will move into him. Allow him to moan and even scream if he feels the need, since either one will keep his breathing regular and release some of the energy building up in him. Screaming, of course, will depend on how soundproof your walls are. A gag will muffle the screams but still allow the release of some sound as well as the pent-up energy.

Did he like it? Unfortunately, he may not have a raging hard-on during anal play or stimulation even if he likes it a great deal. So read his body language. Is he breathing heavily, panting? Look at his face. Is it screwed up in pleasure; is his mouth hanging open? Is he thrusting his hips up, as if seeking more? These are good signs when you are lacking any firmer evidence. Or else just ask him!

Of prime importance is the angle of entry into the rectum. The rectum is a tube but not a straight one and furthermore, the angle of entry varies from person to person. There are not many nerve endings inside the rectum but the tissue there is delicate and tears easily. Inside the anus, the lower rectum tilts forward toward the navel then back again toward the tailbone. Driving anything in on a forward rather than straight-up angle is bound to be overly painful and could tear or damage sensitive tissue. Go slowly and carefully. If he says stop or his safe word, stop immediately. Do not try to withdraw or proceed until you have given him time to relax and his body to adjust.

If he likes your finger, try two. Remember to keep everything lubricated, and as you feel him relax more and more, you can gradually increase your stroke. If anal play turns both of you on, and you would like to try bigger and better things, a butt plug would be a nice addition to your growing collection. There is an almost bewildering array of anal toys and you can be guided by personal preference as well as what is best and safe.

Available in everything from hard plastic to soft vinyl, in fleshy pink, jet black, or all the neon colors of the rainbow, the most common butt plug shape is a cone with a flat bottom that narrows before flaring to its maximum circumference, then tapers off at the top. The soft plastic ones are the safest and most pleasurable to use for anal entry. Anal toys are narrower at the tip and narrow again near the base. The cone shape is what keeps the plug inside. Most adult stores carry three sizes: small for the beginner, medium for the more enthusiastic, and too big. The too-big ones resemble pyramids and have been known to reduce potential recipients to either tears or uncontrollable laughter. Catalogues have a much better selection, offering not only stationary butt plugs but ones that vibrate, inflate, or both.

Start him with the smallest butt plug even if you have given him more than one finger. The feeling of a soft, warm finger and even a small butt plug is very different and he needs time to get used to it. The idea is to penetrate him slowly with the least amount of pain so you can continue to stretch him to make subsequent excursions easier. Then you can gradually increase him to the medium size. I would suggest covering your anal toys with condoms if for no other reason than to make it easier to clean them. Never put anything with sharp or rough edges into the rectum.

In "Ice," I promised to tell you a tiny torture to inflict upon his rectum. Take an ice cube and pass it back and forth under running water until all sharp edges are melted. Then insert the ice cube into the anus just far enough to pass the muscles but not slip inside. Although you will "see" a reaction in less than ten seconds, hold the ice cube inside him for about twenty-five seconds and then take it out. It doesn't hurt but the sensation is unbelievable. Try it on yourself if you are curious. I did. It will take a few minutes for his skin to thaw out before you can reinsert it—if he will let you!

Some people worry, even panic, about inserted items getting lost in the rectum. Don't. This area was made to empty itself out, so take a magazine and sit a spell before you go running off to the emergency room.

~ 14 ~

Sensory Deprivation

Sensory Deprivation is an exercise in isolation. By depriving him of his sight, hearing, and speech, you are releasing him from sexual responsibility. Sensory deprivation is the official term for the more familiar acts we call gagging, blindfolding, and earplugging. During a sensory deprivation experience with the noise, sight, and weight of the world lifted from the bound one's shoulders, he is able to float free in the eroticism of the scene, secure in the knowledge he is looked after by his mistress.

Other devices would include different types of facial hoods, but that is for the Perverati since many hoods can be dangerous. Hoods are also referred to as "facial restraints." Four of our five senses happen in our heads and are put out of commission when a hood is donned. For the beginner, this sudden loss can be terribly overwhelming. This blockage or interference can be very disorienting and may lead to panic. So, for the time being, stay away from facial restraints. He can also be deprived of his fifth sense, touch. Straightjackets, in leather or canvas, restrain the hands, arms, and upper body of the bound one. I find this is very sensual but it does take some getting used to. If you would like to try a straightjacket on him, make sure it is on his list, too!

As with many other aspects of D&S, sensory deprivation is usually performed in conjunction with another fetish. Bound and blindfolded, gagged and bound, gagged and dressed, bound, gagged, plugged, and blindfolded. The mix is endless and naturally differs for each one.

Blindfolds

Blindfolding is the most common form of sensory deprivation, and blindfolds are wonderful toys for beginners. When I plan on depriving him of more than one sense, I always deprive him of his sight first. This is a very powerful weapon in the mistress's arsenal. Depriving him of his sight heightens all of his other senses. The scent of your perfume intensifies and diminishes as you pass by him. The click of your heels becomes a thunderclap to his ears. Touch him without warning and see him jump, hear him gasp.

I love to combine a blindfold and earplugs with some form of bondage and corporal punishment, After he has assumed his position and paid me the proper homage due a goddess, I simply order him into the bedroom. Think of how wonderful it will feel, ladies, to order him to do something and not have him ask why.

I let him wait there for me a few seconds. As I walk in, I am already telling him how I want him positioned on the bed. Faceup or down, spread-eagled or arms and legs together, or legs together and arms apart, or even arms together and legs apart. Anything I want or just the first words out of my mouth, it's so nice to have him eagerly awaiting my every command. And obeying it.

Tonight, I select the spread-eagle, faceup variation. None of the equipment I need to act out the fantasy is visible. To impress his helplessness upon him, I order him into position on the bed and make him wait there while I pull out the first item. Actually, all I had to do was pull the rope ends out from under the bed. I had tied them to the metal bed frame earlier. Lucky you if you have a four-poster bed or brass headboard.

For some reason, I prefer to tie his wrists before his ankles. Maybe it's from the old "bound hand and foot" cliché but that's what I usually do. My feeling is he will feel more helpless sooner if I deprive him of his hands first.

There he is, bound hand and foot to the bed, your helpless prisoner. Now that he has watched and cooperated in his own captivity it's the time to deprive him of his sight. Your wardrobe contains many things you can use to blindfold him. Do you have a silk scarf, or stockings?

Maybe a sleep mask? Then you have a blindfold. I use a regular black satin sleep mask even though there are dozens of varieties of leather masks available. Unless he has a fetish for leather or leather masks, anything that obliterates his vision will work just fine.

Watch his face as you cover his eyes. As soon as his sight is gone, you will notice a change in the visible half of his face. My slave's jaw tends to slacken a little, and his mouth looks more vulnerable than when he has his sight. When he is fully under, he works his lower jaw back and forth, licking his lips frequently. With time, you will notice he has the same reaction each time you blindfold him.

So now you have him bound hand and foot to the bed and the blindfold is in place. What next? Make some noise. Not loud noises but little ones. Open a drawer and take something out of it, something you want to use on him. If that makes a noise, make it. Open the closet and take out your whip or a belt. (No metal tipped belts, please.) Then be really quiet for a little while before you make another sound. Watch him flinch or jump when you do. This will heighten the suspense and add to your mystery.

Gags

Gags are popular items to increase feelings of helplessness but also to stop a person from talking and that is where the danger lies. Of the three items covered here, only this one can present a danger to your partner. The most popular, "the ball gag," is the one you've seen in bondage photos everywhere. It's usually red or black and has buckles or a strap of some other fastening device running out of either side to tie behind his head. Although considered to be very sexy as well as functional, this is the type of gag that can flood your partner's mouth with saliva and cause him to choke. The ball gag inhibits his swallowing by holding his mouth open, which seems to cause him to make more saliva. But he can't swallow because his mouth is being held open . . . this is where the danger comes in. And *never* gag anyone who has a stuffy nose or a cold, trouble breathing, or a cough!

However, if he is a chatterbox, you can gag him safely and effectively with one of your scarves, stockings or even a nice piece of rope.

Tie a large double or triple knot in the center of the chosen item then tie it behind or on the side of his head. If you are using rope, try tying the ends in his mouth like part of the "gag." Try not to use your favorite silk scarf for gagging. Silk, or nylon hosiery, tends to slip and pull the knots very tight so tight you can't untie them to free him. You may have to use your scissors to release him, thereby ruining your scarf.

Put the knot in his mouth and tie the ends behind his head. Or, on the side of his head if you are going to have him lie down. The fabric will soak up his saliva. Instant gag. Be creative. Use your panties, or his. If he is a foot worshiper, your stockings will do just fine. So will your foot!

Formal gags include the "bit" or "bar" gag which is like the bit in a horse's bridle and much less harsh on the sub's mouth than a ball gag. A pipe gag is a set of leather straps connected to an open section of pipe which goes in the mouth, holding it open. Talking is inhibited but the mouth is available for other uses.

One slave of mine wouldn't allow me to gag him but he talked incessantly. And he drove me crazy with all his chattering. So I went into a pet shop looking for a small dog's ball one he could hold in his teeth but didn't need to be tied to his head. He had been gagged and tortured as a prisoner of war so gagging was a horrifying experience for him. But, if he yakked on and on about nothing at his captors the way he yakked at me, I can't blame them for gagging him.

The salesperson in the pet shop couldn't keep his eyes off me as I tried one size ball after another in my mouth. Finally I found one that was just right. It even came in purple. Instant gag not attached to the head. I made him fetch it then didn't take it from him, just let him sit there with it in his mouth. A moment's peace, at last!

Since your slave's mouth is out of commission, you will have to devise some "safe" signal to replace the "safe" word he cannot utter. Some people say three emphatic grunts is a good signal, but the dom had better hear those grunts and fast! I think giving the gagged one something to hold: a red bandana to wave, a ball to drop, a feather so he can wave it if his hands are free, is more reliable. An emphatic left-right head shake which you must constantly be on the alert for will suffice as a safe signal if his hands are not free. You can work out the signals for yourselves, but don't forget to do it.

Earplugs

Lastly, he's ready to be deprived of his hearing. The ears are often over-looked as an erotic zone except for nuzzling. Well, we're not going to nuzzle here, or maybe not yet. The earplugs that are the safest are the soft, almost waxy ones that conform to the shape of the ear. Earplugs will not render him deaf to all sound but they do tune out the noise you will be making. By this time, your slave should be trembling with anticipation.

Now you have him where you want him. At your mercy, your bound, naked slave. What do you do with him? First, I would suggest a stim-ulus, maybe tweak his nipples. Men's nipples are very sensitive. If you are imaginative, in low, cool tones, tell him a story, if he's not wearing earplugs, of course! Preferably one about what you are going to do to him. You could swish a feather back and forth across his prone, naked flesh. A leather glove, a fur mitt, the ends of your hair, something cool or cold, or something he can't identify will also serve to sensitize him and bolster your authority over him. This should give you a good feel-ing of empowerment. Remember, when he's bound and deprived of his senses everything you do to him will be enhanced.

～ 15 ～

Slaves and Slave Training

Within the D&S community there is contention over the use of "slave" versus "submissive." Some think the word "slave" is degrading, with its connotations of ownership and less-than-human principles. These people prefer to be called "submissives." The others love to be called "slave" for those very reasons! Some think of themselves as the mistress's slave, not her submissive, because being a "slave boy" or a "boy toy," with its sexual implications and connotations, is more erotic and romantic. Although some prefer the word "slave," they have no real objection to being called submissive because, used as a verb, that's what they are being. So here I will use the two words, as nouns, interchangeably. But there is an important difference between a masochistic state and a submissive one. The vanilla world uses "slave" and "masochist" to denote the one and the same emotional state.

A masochist desires, loves, craves, seeks out pain of a physical or emotional nature. The slave is on a different level emotionally. His desire is to please the mistress in whatever way she desires. He wants to be her "slave" in the literal sense. The masochist may have little or no desire to play the submissive; the submissive may have few or no masochistic tendencies.

The Sexual Slave

The slave's fantasy of surrendering control of his life, even temporarily, to another person has an undeniable allure. Many men who want to be

slaves have high-powered, stressful careers, controlling the fate and for-
tunes of others on a daily basis. He is out there doing battle in the real
world every day. Playing the slave and surrendering control is an exhil-
arating, heady experience for him. And it may be the first time in his
life he has surrendered that control. Consenting to being a slave gives
him a chance to turn himself inside out and explore his "dark side." The
consent itself is very sexy and a powerful aphrodisiac for him. Hearing
himself say out loud for the first time, "Yes, I will serve you, I will give
you my body to use for your pleasure, I am your slave," excites him.
And soon those words become an intoxicatingly seductive mantra. It
exemplifies one of the exciting things about being a sexual slave: it
allows him to fulfill his fantasies without guilt. In the case of the slave,
he has no choice but to obey; he is not responsible for his sexuality
because he has given the reins of control over to someone else. Your
acceptance of his fantasy, in particular of being a "slave," gives him permission to act the fantasy out.

It is important for you to understand what he is feeling as a slave,
especially the first few times you play. This may be one of the few times
in his life he is powerless over the direction of it. You are dressed; he is
not. Imagine how it would feel to wear your genitals on the outside of
your body like he wears his. He is feeling quite vulnerable as he entrusts
his well-being to you. You, of course, want to take advantage of this but
be careful not to destroy his self-image in the process.

To abandon himself as a sexual slave is a powerful aphrodisiac for
him. A sexual slave spends his days and nights in a state of constant
anticipatory sexual arousal. Being the slave is provocative, alluring, and
enticing. It provides a healthy emotional outlet for feelings and desires
that would not otherwise be expressed. As your sexual slave, he can surrender to the erotic part of his nature without fear of harm or guilt;
there is no need for him to exercise self-restraint. By pretending that he
has no choice, he can forget that he actually does have one and go as
far as his mind will take him.

Since he is your partner he can trust you not to abuse that surrender.
The intimacy of a D&S relationship built on trust and communication is
almost spiritual. As my wise friend Bob H. once said, "Other people
repress their demons. We harness ours up and take them out for a ride."

Slave Training

In the introduction, we had a dress rehearsal of a play session from start to finish. By now, he knows his positions, one through ten, and can execute each perfectly on command. He has memorized the rules and can even follow them most of the time. Both of you like D&S play and now you want to play some more. You would like to give him some formal training on how to serve or please you on a regular basis. This is not to say that you are going to have what D&Sers call a "24/7/365." That means twenty-four hours a day, seven days a week, three hundred sixty-five days a year. Who could be in role day in and day out? I remember clients who were amazed that I didn't get up in the morning and put my "boots" on.

You know by now that "slave" and "masochist" are not synonymous. Your slave may be one of the many who does not like to be beaten. A slave's deepest desire is to serve you, his mistress. And that could mean anything. Some slaves are very specific in what they like to do while serving. Others will leave it entirely up to you to direct their preparation and activities.

His own preparations are as important as yours; in this case, his personal hygiene. The slave should come to the mistress freshly bathed and shampooed, recently shaven, and deodorized. He should have just brushed his teeth and his tongue. Additionally, his nails should be neatly and smoothly trimmed and if the mistress prefers a particular scent, that cologne should be worn. As he performs his preparations, he should be emotionally readying himself to play, thinking about the playtime and eroticizing it, and making himself fall in love with the idea of being your sexual slave.

The Trial-and-Error Method

Now that he is all squeaky clean and shiny, you need a way to establish what his activities will be. If he has not told you what he has dreamt of doing, you can please yourself or you can use the trial-and-error (T&E) method to determine what he does best. This method is a lot of fun since you can discover things about each other you may not have known prior to your awakening to D&S.

The best way to put the T&E method into effect is to observe him and combine your observations with what you already know about him. Let's say you know he gives a good massage. You may want to train him as a bath slave since the skills needed for massaging and bathing are comparable. One slave I had gave an excellent massage. As a treat one night, I ordered him to give me a bath.

I supervised the filling of the tub, selected the amount and type of bubble bath I wanted and which skin softeners I preferred that night. My slave undressed me as I directed, then he folded my clothes neatly out of the way. Holding my hand, he helped me into the steaming, fragrant tub. I sank down into the luxurious bubbles only to find my bath pillow needing inflating. I instructed him to blow it up for me and reposition it exactly where I wanted it.

Since his massage technique was very good, I assumed he would need very little instruction as to how to give a good bath. Much to my surprise, he needed absolutely no instruction at all! This was the very best bath I had ever had. His style was to hold the soap in his cupped hand and rub it firmly but gently on my skin. Like a combination of massaging and washing at the same time.

I tried to describe this special technique to others who showed an affinity for massage but to no avail. Mr. Bath Slave had it and, much to my chagrin, no amount of instruction from me could impart it to another.

If he is handy around the house, consider setting him to those little tasks he never gets around to doing otherwise. I find this to be particularly endearing when the only thing he is wearing is his tool belt.

If you find he doesn't give good massage and you are handier with the hammer than he is, don't give up. There are still dozens of things you can train him to do. For the foot slave, I would recommend a regimen of shoe and boot maintenance. If he watches with interest as you blow-dry your hair, teach him how to do it for you. Assign him the task of laundering your hand washables. Do you hate to wash windows? Sweep? Vacuum? Dust? Scrub the bathtub? Or the toilet bowl? (If his aim is poor when he tinkles and he tends to get it down the front of the bowl, this will impress upon him to be more careful with his stream.) Washing, waxing, and vacuuming the car also spring to mind.

As does cleaning out his closet, the garage, basement, or shed. Once I sent my slave down the hall to the garbage chute, naked, his long hair streaming out behind him!

The Reward-and-Punishment System

Now that you have established what he does best, how do you train him to do it your way? He is your slave, ladies, you tell him how you want it done. However, it is not always that easy.

Men are hardwired differently from women and maybe some of them *are* from Mars (the planet, not the god of war). Women are the superior sex for a number of reasons. We have internal plumbing, like all advanced models. It is true "God" created man before he created woman but you always make the rough draft before the final masterpiece.

A man is unable to run a house, raise the kids, get the dinner on the table, and have clean clothes for everyone each and every day of the year. He is unable to cope with the everyday world the way a woman does because he doesn't understand it. Men are unable to see the whole picture, think things through from A to Z, and then come up with a plan. You are the one who deserves to be idolized, not him. Show him his proper place in the larger scheme of things. On his knees, before you.

Now that we have had our little pep talk, we'll get back to how to train him. I would recommend combining the trial-and-error method with the reward-and-punishment system of training at first. Simply put, reward for good behavior and punishment for bad. Punishment need not be corporal; it could be the removal of the object of his desire or your attentions and affections. If he is a foot slave, reward him by letting him massage your feet or kiss them. Punish him by withdrawing your feet and forbidding him to touch them. Then tease him with them by touching them yourself and tell him if he had been good, he would be caressing them now. Or, if he is turned on, don't let him come until he has made you come, at least once. That's a very good noncorporal punishment. Later on, we'll discuss an advanced method of slave training called "Planting the Seed."

As I stressed earlier, atmosphere is an important ingredient as you weave your spell. Make sure the room is warm enough for nakedness, light the candles, and get the music going. Give him the prearranged signal that playtime has begun.

Establish beforehand if a whipping, even a light one, is within his limits. If he is not into playing with pain, this would be a symbolic beating more than genuine corporal punishment. A good slave's desire is to please you and if beating him pleases you, he will accept it because it is your wish.

So now you know what he is good at, he is in the position of your choice, ready, willing, and eager to obey your every command. How do you go about training him? Have you ever trained a dog or seen one being trained? The same methods can be adjusted for humans and used beneficially to guide your slave.

Be clear in your instructions to him. This is not the time to be mealymouthed or shy. Speak up, sing out, repeat yourself. Make your desires known. Remember you are in control here. The reason he wants to be your slave is to relinquish control of his life for a specified period of time. He's giving that control to you, take it!

When you assign him a task, supervise him. You've given him the duty of laundering your hand washables. It is safe to assume that he knows absolutely nothing about hand wash and delicate things. Have you ever seen a man sort laundry? Of course not, that's why his white things have a pink tinge. So it is up to you to direct him. Stand next to the sink as he fills it up, point out which soap you want and how much of it he should use. Ask him to repeat it back to you to fix it in his memory. Then oversee the actual washing. Correct him when he makes a mistake. Teach him how to sort your clothes, point out that the label in the garment specifies the washing instructions and they should be followed. If he ruins it, have him replace it for you with something twice as expensive. That should get the point across if nothing else does.

Although many times you have to use the process of elimination to gauge what is a turn-on for him, other times you will hit upon things he likes quite accidentally. Being able to tell if it turns him on is very easy. He's naked! His excitement will be visible to you in the form of an erection, as will his boredom or dissatisfaction.

I was spending a cold winter evening with Cupcake when I stumbled across two new things I could add to our ever-growing repertoire.

He was in his assigned position on his cushion at my feet. This was his home base. He was "at ease" with his hands on the floor on either side of him, his fingers spread apart.

As I rose from my chair on my way to get the candle I use for hot waxing, I stepped rather heavily on his outspread fingers. Realizing what I had done, I turned expecting to see him clutching his fingers in pain. What I saw instead was the special glazed look he gets in his eyes that is reserved for extreme pleasure that I never see at any other time.

After seeing that, naturally I did not apologize for stepping on him when he so obviously liked it. "Oh, was that you? I thought it was too soft to be the floor," I said playfully and went on my merry way. Part of being a mistress means never having to say you are sorry. I could have *meant* to step on his fingers. After all, he *did* like it.

Later on that same evening, when he was again crouched at my feet on his cushion, his own disobedience was the cause of my second discovery. He knows he is not allowed to touch my feet without my express permission. In spite of this, he is still a foot lover and he cannot resist my feet even if it means punishment.

As he rested his face against the toe of my pump, I caught him trying to sneak a kiss on my shoe. I rose in feigned anger to discipline him and didn't realize his lip was wrapped underneath the sole of my shoe. I stepped on his lip! He gasped and moaned in what I could tell was pleasure. When I removed my foot from his mouth, he thanked me for stepping on him! He didn't know it was an accident and not part of his punishment. So I didn't tell him. I just let him think I was wonderful, beautiful and creative, and wasn't he lucky to have me as his mistress?

Planting the Seed

The trial-and-error method is excellent when you want to find out what he is good at but what if you want to do something with him, enact some fantasy or scenario that is erotic to you but he doesn't seem interested in? There is another method of training, more subtle, less hands-on, that D&Sers call "planting the seed." Even city dwellers know that when you plant a seed in fertile soil, it will grow. If you are playing at D&S now, then you know the soil is fertile.

Indubitably discovered by a member of the Perverati, the methodology is beautifully simple. I have used it myself dozens of times and have had it used on me as well. I have even used it on myself! Speak to him of the thing, your fantasy, in loving, sharing words. Don't make it seem you are trying to foist this upon him. Your tone should be more like one of "I know you don't want to do this with me but (sigh) thank you for at least listening to me." Then romanticize the hell out of the thing. Use your softest, most beguiling tone of voice; make him feel as if you are speaking from your secret heart much in the way he spoke to you. Don't do anything else and most of all, don't rush things. Just talk lovingly of it, even a little wistfully if you like, now and then.

And mark my words, as sure as welts follow cane marks, he will come to *you* and begin to talk of the thing in a romantic, slave-speech fashion. What happens is that he begins to fantasize on the thing himself, slowly at first, maybe once or twice the day after you mention it. As he does that, he finds that bits and pieces of the fantasy are starting to appeal to him. So he dwells on those and romanticizes them. But those bits and pieces cannot exist in fantasy limbo; they need a scenario to go around them. And here he has one, complete with a suitable partner, the fantasy you spoke to him of only a short time ago. Often the thing that frightens the slave the most will ultimately be the thing that turns him on the most. He will beg you to enact this fantasy with him, be that person for him. The seed you planted took root and grew into a new experience for both of you.

Punishment

What if his service is unsatisfactory? We have already established that some slaves do not want to be beaten as punishment so you will have to find other ways to discipline them. If your partner does not want to receive a beating as punishment, I would suggest withholding sexual release. Make sure he is good and hard but *do not* let him come until he has pleased you. Again, he is a slave—he is not allowed to come without your permission.

Having his orgasm controlled by you is highly erotic for the submissive. It enforces his fantasy of being totally subject to the whims of another, or his fantasy of being a sex toy, or his fantasy of being an object, and many another fantasy, too. We women are lucky in that our arousal is hard to detect with the naked eye. Only the skilled male or master will notice that our nipples change color when we are aroused, or that our mons venus swells and reddens in anticipation, among other things. But his! His is plainly visible and that visibility can be used to tease and torment him. One of my favorite games to play with his orgasm is to have him come on my command. This first involves a soliloquy about what good service I have received or how pleased I am by his progress. This is the signal that I want him to come soon so he can "gear up" and then there is a "count," usually to ten. Sometimes we don't make it to ten but that's all right.

When you punish him is entirely up to you. And it also depends on the kind of punishment he is going to receive at your hands. If corporal punishment is in order, you can punish him as soon as he commits the infraction or you can save it all up and punish him at the end of the session. If you will not be beating him, I suggest you punish him right after the infraction has been committed.

If corporal punishment is in order, you have many choices as to when you can give him his just desserts. You may want to give him ten lashes or spanks or strokes as soon as he displeases you. Or you may want him to keep a running tally of all the lashes you owe him to be administered at the end of the session. Or you can combine these two and punish him during and after the session. Or at the start of the session to remind him of things to come or what he can expect if he disobeys. A popular task for the mistress to assign the slave to perform is to count out each stroke as he receives it. As in, "One, Mistress Claudia, thank you!." Or to ask you for the next stroke, "One, Mistress Claudia, may I have another?" You can combine the two but it takes a long time to say both of them together, rendering the strokes too far apart. And if he says them too fast, it renders the beauty of his words useless as he sputters to get them out before the next stroke lands.

If you are punishing him at the finale of the session, it may help to reiterate what you are punishing him for. You could point out that these ten strokes are for this infraction and these ten are for that. Having him count out each stroke for you before you land it impresses his disobedience and its ultimate outcome in his mind.

If you are not punishing him corporally, then I would again suggest you punish him immediately after the infraction occurs. Like training a puppy, it does no good to put your foot back in your shoe two hours after he has kissed your arch without permission.

One of the hardest aspects of slave training is keeping things consistent yet different and interesting. Mistressing can be hard work with what D&Sers call a "do-me-queen." This slave gives you nothing, just lies there and wants it all to be done to him. Even with a communicative slave, D&S involves some work. And, slaves generally do not realize how hard it is to be the mistress. You have to keep him occupied each and every minute during playtime as well as comport yourself with the appropriate attitude while you are doing it. All he has to do is sit there, or kneel there, and await your command. You have to think up the commands, assess his performance of them, and then correct and/or discipline him. This can be especially trying if you yourself have had a hard day at the office or are tired and he is not cooperating fully.

Empowerment

Many a dominant enjoys asking her slave certain questions to elicit specified answers. These are called "ritualized questions and answers" and the answers are designed to empower you as the mistress when asked of your slave. I don't feel the exact question is that important, although some do. Too many rules make the game no fun and the question that has the most empowering answer for you is the right one. You may want to ask him who he is: "I am your slave, Mistress." Or what he will do to please you: "I will do anything you command, Mistress." Or perhaps: "I live only to please you, Mistress." Other dominants favor ritualized commands, such as "present," when ordering the slave to assume a pre-arranged punishment position.

You will need some way of knowing whether what you have commanded is distasteful to him, or unnecessary. Let's say he has brought you a snack or beverage at your demand. You offer him some of it and he doesn't want any. He should never say "No," or even "No, thank you,

Mistress." If he doesn't want any, his response to you could be something like, "Not only if it pleases you, Mistress." The negative "not" makes his preference clear; many ritualized responses seem nonsensical when spoken out of context. On the other hand, if he does want it, he could say "If it pleases you, Mistress."

There are subtle ways you can make your dominant side apparent even to a nonbeliever. One evening I went to a large D&S party hosted by a mistress who was well known in the Northeast. Her home was out of the city so we met at a central location and piled into whatever cars were available to us. I was in the back seat of the "smokers' car," along with an Austrian dominatrix and a very handsome male on the fringe of the scene. The front seat was claimed by the submissive driver and a woman who claimed to have a "bad back." The handsome male was a guest of this woman.

On the ride to the party, my sister-in-domination got into a disagreement with the male. He was saying there was no such thing as a naturally dominant woman, it was all an act to make a woman feel better, and that she was lucky the man went along with it, and so forth along those lines. The woman, who was quite charming, was doing her best not to start an argument with him in such closed surroundings. She knew it would be unpleasant for the rest of us, as we were five people in a four-seater car.

She gracefully demurred, possibly to let him think he had won the battle. But I knew better. She may have conceded the battle, but the war had just barely begun. Once inside, she went out of her way to charm him in a delightfully feminine way, and in a short time had him at her side awaiting her every word. But those words were actually commands.

She couched her commands to sound like polite requests of the type a woman would usually give her man at a party. Another drink, an ashtray, a cocktail napkin, a light for her cigarette, another hors d'oeuvre. What was so wonderful was the way that she did it. She would ask for another drink, he would return with it. After he was reseated on a hassock (in a lower position than hers) and looked comfortable, she would find something wrong with the way he executed his last errand. She did this in the sweetest way, with a smile and kindly tone, making him feel remiss in his duty to her. Upon which, he would literally spring up to attend to the forgotten napkin or insufficient quantity of ice.

She knew that I knew she was enforcing a subtle type of slave training on him, and every time she sent him charging off to see to her needs, she and I would start to laugh as soon as he was out of earshot. She must have sent him off on a good dozen errands, some of them for me, and he still hadn't caught on. I could see what she was doing to him but he couldn't!

Of course, I did not interfere with this little enactment. That would have been in bad taste since the initial disagreement was between my lady friend and the guy. If a lesson was to be taught, it was only right that she be the teacher.

After more than an hour of this had passed, she turned to him and said, "You have just been the slave of two mistresses for over one hour. You served us, you ran to fulfill our every command, and showed remorse when it was not to our satisfaction. Have you changed your mind about dominant women?" His face turned bright red, his jaw open and shut several times, making him look like a landed fish, and then he did an about-face and stomped off into the crowd.

I was fairly new to letting my real dominant self out when this happened, and I was very impressed with the way my Austrian sister-in-domination handled this recalcitrant male. It taught me that a woman doesn't have to raise her voice or use strong-arm tactics to dominate a man. Her own feminine wiles combined with her fine, keen mind will win out over the "stronger" sex most every time.

Slave Contracts

The thought of signing a slave contract is a hot fantasy. Having a piece of paper that signs away your rights to your body and makes you chattel fuels many a submissive fantasy fire on a cold night. In a serious or committed D&S relationship, both of you may wish to set out your limits, goals, obligations, and expectations in an oral or written contract. Of course, these "contracts" have no force in law but they do carry some responsibilities.

Before signing a slave contract, stop and think about, and reread each and everything that has been written. Please know that for some, committing those ideas and fantasies to paper, and giving the top full permission to act them out on and with the bottom, is a true and valid contract that they expect to be honored. So give each word, each phrase careful consideration before writing it down. Is he ready to relinquish his safe word, to submit without knowing what is going to happen to him? Is he ready to trust you fully and completely like he has trusted no other in his life? Does he think you are intelligent and sensitive enough to know when he needs to work and not to play? If you have said, Yes, Yes, and Yes, then sign your name and seal it with a fresh lipstick kiss.

Ideally the Mistress/Slave Contract is created together and defines the obligations, aspirations, and rights of both parties. Writing this contract together will help you define your relationship more clearly and enhance your communication skills. The contract should be realistic in scope; it does not exist just to turn you on. It represents a serious commitment and should be taken seriously.

But in the meantime, don't hesitate to use it as a hot fantasy!

∼ 16 ∼

Water Sports

Golden Showers

The mistress's nectar, golden stream, or yellow ambrosia, whatever you choose to call it, the rite of golden showers is often misunderstood by the uninitiated. Most people think of golden showers as something the slave wants done in his mouth so he can drink it. That is not always the case.

The most common form of a golden shower has nothing to do with drinking urine at all. A man with voyeuristic tendencies often wants to be in the bathroom while the mistress is relieving herself of her golden stream. If the mistress is able (some ladies are pee-shy and can't go when someone else is in the room), then the ultimate treat for this man would be to watch her as she tinkles. The lady would sit down to do her business in her normal manner. He would then peek between the toilet seat and bowl or look between her parted thighs to watch her stream as it leaves her body. This activity can be very cute and endearing since the man is often tickled to death about what he has seen. D&S players call this "drinking fresh from the fountain."

The first man who shared this fantasy with me was absolutely delighted when I responded positively to his request. According to him, I was the first lady to have ever agreed to let him watch and he was thrilled. I thought it was cute and harmless and I had to go really badly anyway so why not?

So I sat down with my knees apart and let him crawl between my legs so he could peek between the two seats. When he saw I had no problem relieving myself in front of him, he became bolder and asked me if I could "go a little slower." I went a little slower; emboldened by my new-found "control", I went really hard, then I stopped completely, then I let a little more out. He realized I was controlling my stream for his benefit and stimulation and began egging me on. "Can you just go a few drops?" I complied. "Okay, fast now." Again I complied. "Can you make it start and stop and start again?" I could do that too, so I did. Hey, this was fun for both of us and no one *drank* anything, except for me. I had quite a few glasses of water to enhance his viewing pleasure.

And I will never forget the first time I gave Mickey a golden shower. We were showering together, soaping each other up and generally fooling around when I started to become amorous. I slithered up to Mickey, wrapped my arms around his neck and stuck my tongue down his throat. Then I pulled his thigh right up between my thighs. I began to rub my pussy on him, knowing I had to tinkle, and when the time was right, I let loose down his leg. It took him a few seconds to realize all the water in the shower was not coming from the faucet but that some of it was coming from me.

"Are you peeing on me?" "Yes." Being Mickey, he started to laugh and called me a slithery, slippery wee-wee sneak. Then he asked if he got a turn. Of course he did, I replied, he could "go" any place below my waist. Since I have a nice round bottom, he chose it as his target. It did take him a few extra seconds to get it started but when it did start, there was no stopping him. He was making figure eights on my cheeks; he was scripting out his initials; he was drawing tic-tac-toe boards; in other words, he really got into it. I have since come to learn that many women have showered their men in the same playful manner.

With clients, I have given many golden showers with excellent results. Not that I slithered up to the client in the shower and stuck my tongue in his mouth. Mickey was my lover and we played together all the time. With clients, the scene was quite a bit different and no touching was involved.

The standard scenario with a client would usually include humiliation during the session as well as the golden shower at the finale of the session. One client liked me to "tank" up in front of him and keep up a constant conversation about how I was just recycling this water to use on him later. Another client liked to hear "pee-pee stories" while I filled up in front of him. I would relate tales of peeing behind a bush, in a parking lot, on the beach, over a log, all sorts of public places, narrowly missing detection by the people all around me.

At the finale, the slave would climb into the bathtub and lie almost flat. Still dressed, I would stand with one foot on each side of the top of the tub and yank my panties to the side. Then I would relieve myself on his genitals, teasing him by starting and stopping myself, or letting a few drops come out and no more, until he begged for it. My aim got to be so good, I could direct my stream at one of his balls, or pee only on the tip of his cock! Occasionally, I would urinate into a carafe and threaten him with it as a punishment drink.

There are members of the Perverati who do drink the golden nectar, however.

Last March, I attended the Tenth Annual Sex Maniacs Ball in London. I wore a floor-length leather halter dress that contained yards of leather and covered absolutely nothing. The ballroom and exhibition rooms were well heated but the bathroom was an arctic zone. And, there were a dozen ladies ahead of me. It was too cold and I had waited until the last minute and now couldn't wait anymore. I was about to pee in my dress. Then I remembered seeing people come away from the bar with tall neon-colored plastic glasses. If I could find one of those . . . !

I did. I grabbed it and trotted back to the table where my friends were sitting. I made my way around to the back of the table, near the wall. I hoisted my dress up, squatted and positioned the cup between my legs. A loud sigh of relief escaped me in a rare moment of silence in an otherwise noisy place. In other words, just then the damn music stopped (don't you just hate when that happens?) and everyone for a twenty-foot radius heard me. The entire table and then some turned to look at me but at that point I had to go so bad I didn't care! It felt so good I just smiled and kept on peeing. When I was finished, I reached in my bag and took out a wet-wipe and cleaned myself. This broke them up. I sometimes carry them in my bag but I'm sure these people thought I had them with me because I peed so often in glasses! Then I carefully placed the glass to the side so I wouldn't spill it when I stood.

As I rose, a gray-haired, blue-eyed old gentleman approached and said enthusiastically, "There are plenty here that would like to drink that, you know, Mistress. Would you like me to find you one?" I very politely declined his, er, generous offer.

Knowing it is not sanitary to drink anyone's urine but your own, I question the safety of this fetish. The means of ingestion vary from the standing up method described earlier to urinating in a glass and presenting it to him, to a funnel attached to a tube that he holds in his mouth. Between you and me, I doubt your man is going to ask for this pleasure but you never know!

Enemas

There are probably thousands who love enemas but are ashamed to come clean about it. Others run screaming at the mere mention of the word. Why? The idea of someone invading your anus with a nozzle attached to a hose hooked up to a bag of water about to be emptied into your belly, for the vast majority, is not erotic. But enemas have been with us a very long time. Ancient Egyptians purged their bellies with nozzles carved like the beaks of ibis; ancient burial sites of priests in Central and upper South America revealed enema bags which archaeologists believe were used by the priests to introduce trance-inducing drugs into their body by the anal canal. The ancient Greeks purged; Chaucer knew of purges; so did the court of Louis XIV. Many people administer enemas without the eroticism of it crossing their minds. Yet enemas play a special role in a D&S relationship.

For the receiver in a D&S relationship, an enema is a humbling affair, and leaves no doubt as to who is in control. The setting of the D&S enema scene exemplifies the dominant's power in no uncertain terms. For many there is role-playing involved in the enema; for some there is not. The roles assumed could be nurse/patient, or older relative/child. In the mistress/slave scenario, the slave is forced to accept an enema as punishment, discipline, humiliation, or in preparation for anal play. But no matter what the scenario, the dominant's power is explicit.

The slave is nude while the dominant remains dressed. Since the scene often takes place in the bathroom, the naked slave can be made to lie in the tub, sit over the end of the tub, or can assume one or two humiliating positions on the floor. The slave can be made to bend over at the waist and grasp the side of the tub; kneel with his shoulders on the floor and his hips in the air; or lie on his left side, knees slightly drawn up to the chest. The slave's anus and genitals are exposed to the dominant's view and are available for her amusement.

After inserting the nozzle, the top controls the flow of water into the rectum. Some use the Bardex or the double Bardex instead of a regular tube or nozzle that can slip out. In the single Bardex, the Bardex is inflated inside the anus with a small pump to prevent the nozzle from slipping. In the double Bardex, there are two ballooning sections. One inflates inside the body and the other just outside the anus. The slave presents his bottom to his mistress; she fills him with water or enema solution then often inserts a butt plug so that he may not relieve himself without her permission. In a D&S scenario, this is an emotionally charged situation. The dom may choose not to leave the bathroom while he releases; this can be deeply humiliating and as such, a source of sexual excitement. It also impresses upon the slave his helplessness. Not even his bowels are his to control!

Giving an enema isn't difficult but there are some things you should know. The tissues inside the rectum are very delicate and the nozzle or tube should be well lubricated before entry. It's best to use warm water, never hot or cold. Some people experiment with wine or alcohol enemas but I don't believe these are safe so stick with tap water. Absorption through the anal passage is very quick; some people are allergic to sulfites, others have a very low tolerance for alcohol.

The enema bag should be about two feet above the anus so that the flow in is gentle. Use your head when you fill the bag—it shouldn't be full to bursting, and the quantity of water should match the size of the person. A small person would need less water than a larger one. Make sure the hose is full before you begin to enemate him by releasing the clip and letting the air clear the line. This will stop the excess air from being forced into his bowels. The water should flow freely from the nozzle before you insert it. Then you can control the flow by the clip on the hose or tube or by pinching it with your fingers. You, or he, will need to hold the tube in place as muscle contractions can make it slip out. This is where the Bardex comes in handy. He may need for you to pause now and then so he can absorb your gift to him. Be ready to stop the flow if he says "pause" or starts to cramp or leak. If he cramps, you are giving it to him too fast.

When the bag is empty, clamp it off immediately as, again, you do not want to let air inside of him. Be careful not to change the angle of the tube as you withdraw it.

For some, forced retention is an erotic turn-on. Some like to be plugged to add to that full feeling. Others like to be humiliated further. What does he have to do before he can evacuate himself? Give you head until you come? Beg?

Whether or not you stay in the bathroom when he releases is entirely up to you. Some slaves find it thrillingly humiliating to relieve themselves in front of the dominant, others don't. A helpful hint: since the smells associated with this activity are not always pleasant, a scented candle or stick of incense will return your home to its fragrant, sexy state.

~ 17 ~

Bits and Pieces

Bits and pieces is a London expression that can mean many things depending on the context. "Do you have your bits and pieces?" can mean all of your little things: your purse, coat, umbrella, and satchel. Or it can simply mean "everything you need" to get you where you are going: the keys, the address, the invitation. Alternatively, it can be used as a catch-all phrase to denote a bunch of odds and ends that are important but uncategorized. Here I use "bits and pieces" in the catch-all sense: I want to talk about these very titillating and exotic practices because some of them are very visible around us and others are hot fantasies that have lurked in dark corners for too long. But, I don't want to mix the bits and pieces in with the rest of the information because each and every one of them is in the realm of the Perverati.

The information in the following subheads is true exotica and not to be undertaken under any circumstances. I have included it because I am sure many of you are curious about the fantasies, or have questions about them, and I felt I would be remiss in omitting them.

Body Modification

I wonder if the mother who pierces her child's ears, or the dancer who has breast enlargement or reduction, or the actor who pumps iron realize that they are practicing one of humankind's oldest forms self-adornment: body modification.

189

Archaeological evidence for this abounds from all corners of the world. From South America to China, for reasons magical or spiritual, ranging from religious ritual circumcision to piercings for heightened sexual arousal, body modification is practiced universally. Tattoos, enlarged earlobes, elongated necks, cephalic deformation (changing the skull's shape during infancy), corsetted waists, bound feet, patterns burnt or cut into the skin, piercings, brandings, and special cosmetics to enhance your this or that—little on the human body has been left untouched down through the centuries.

Permanent Piercings

Nothing startles a blue-haired granny more than a young person with exotic piercings in their face. Richard Symington, who made millions after having invented Muzak, is considered the "father of the modern rebirth of piercing." Symington helped to organize a group of piercing enthusiasts, among them Jim Ward, who later founded the Gauntlet, the world's best known piercing salon.

The consensus in the D&S scene is that piercings of the erogenous zones heighten sexual pleasure for both the pierced one and their partner. For the submissive, the piercing may indicate ownership or erotic servitude. For the dominant, to order a piercing for her submissive (I would not suggest you do this yourself—go to a professional piercing salon) is a power trip since she is altering his body permanently.

People have tried to pierce just about every part of their bodies but the parts that lend themselves best to being pierced are the parts that protrude. The most common piercings are of the ear, nose (nostril), tongue, lips, nipple, navel, and different parts of the genitalia depending, of course, on your sex.

Men have more of a selection in genital piercings than women do and it is no surprise. Piercings *do* go best on protrusions; and they have more of them than we do. The most common piercing for a man is a "PA" or "Prince Albert." The PA is one of the fastest healing piercings, taking only twelve to eighteen months. This is a ring placed through the urethra and glans. It feels absolutely incredible to have sex with a man who has this piercing. If he is not very well-endowed, this ring will sure-ly make up for what's lacking!

There are many more penis piercing styles that are almost as sexy as the "PA" and feel just as good. The barbell or labret "ampallang" which transects the glans horizontally above the urethra is very popular. This is also one of the longest healing ones, taking at least two years to heal depending on the type of jewelry used. For some the healing time may be as long as four years. The ampallang is also used in combination with a dydoe.

The dydoe is inserted on either or both sides of the glans. It is often combined with a PA or ampallang or the penis is dydoe'd in triplicate. The dydoe takes at least one year to heal, if not more. Male genital pierc-ings in the penis are almost always used for heightened sexual arousal of both the man and the woman.

Female genital piercings are limited to the inner and outer labia, the clitoris and the clitoral hood. Labia piercings are usually done in multi-ples: one or two for each inner or outer lip. In olden days labia rings were used to enforce chastity. This was much kinder than sewing the poor woman closed until she found a husband and married.

Piercing the clitoris or the clitoral hood are the most difficult ones because of the enormous number of nerve endings there. Hood and clit piercings are for those who enjoy intense erotic stimulation and have eight to twelve months to wait for it to be completely healed. All per-manent piercings should be done professionally. Follow the cleaning instructions to the letter and follow all cautions provided by the salon. Do not touch the piercing with your hands unless you've washed them first. Do not swim in a public pool, use a hot tub, or go in an ocean, lake, or any other body of water except your own bathtub. Avoid letting someone else who didn't wash their hands touch the piercing. *Never use jewelry from another part of your body in your piercings.* Earrings do not work as nipple rings—only as earrings!

Yours truly got stung by the piercing bee one day and ran out and got her tongue pierced. I was really excited about the idea, especially since the piercer made "house calls" and I could have a little hen party in celebration. I told the piercer I was allergic to surgical steel and couldn't wear it in my ears. What did he suggest for my tongue? Surgical steel, of course. Assuring me that my tongue was different than other skin and that there were more acids in the mouth, he said surgical steel would be fine. I believed him.

Two weeks later when my tongue was supposed to be healed enough to change the large training labret to the proper size for my mouth, my tongue was still a swollen, flapping, uncontrollable piece of cartiledge and tender to the touch. Additionally, I began to have salivation problems. Either my mouth was so dry my lips were sticking to my teeth or I was drooling. Lovely! And now it sounded like I had a speech impediment. I lost five pounds because I could only eat things I didn't have to manipulate with my tongue. I always carried Listerine and a bottle of water with me even to the nightclub; I followed all the cleaning and care instructions. When he pulled the large labret out to replace it with the smaller one, the hole on the bottom closed up with pus from an infection. We were unable to replace the labret and at that point I decided to let it heal. It was infected and a ball of scar tissue or something else I didn't want to know about came out of it. About four days later it was fine. If I ever get any more piercings, I'm sure they will be joining the others in twelve karat or fourteen karat gold—in my ears!

Play Piercings

If you want to play with needles, this is the way to do it. Play piercings are temporary and although done with sterile needles, they do not leave any scars or marks. Hypodermic needles are usually used and only pierce the upper layers of skin. No jewelry is inserted into the piercing so after the needle is removed the hole closes up and heals. Play piercings are always performed in an erotic setting and may be a form of punishment or a symbol of servitude or ownership. Even though these are temporary and not permanent, play piercings are not done casually, as all penetration of the skin involves potential risk and requires caution.

The needles can be left in place for short periods of time. The more artistic dominants into needle play arrange them in patterns or combine them with silvery thin elastic bands stretched to hook onto door jambs to create winged angels of pain. Some dominants control the sub's movements with the needles and bands like a puppeteer controls a marionette.

Permanent Tattoos

I have wanted a tattoo ever since I saw the star my next door neighbor's mother had on her arm. A tiny little twinkler, she often wore a Band-Aid over it and told me she was sorry she had gotten it. I still thought it was romantic and lovely.

But I have never gotten a permanent tatoo. Maybe I have never been ready to make that kind of commitment to something permanently tattooed on my body. Depending on where your tattoo is and what it depicts, your lifestyle becomes that of your tattoo and announces what you think you are to all and sundry.

Tattooing was condemned in the Old Testament but Egyptian mummies dating from 2000 B.C. have been found bearing tattoos. Some cultures tattoo for glory, others for shame; some for decoration and others for identification. Not until the West got a hold of tattooing did its meaning take on a sinister side: the tattooing of slaves and criminals for identification. In America, tattooing has seized a foothold in subcultures and countercultures. Bikers use tattoos to denote their membership in an elite subculture and signify their outlaw status.

Today tattoos are no longer the symbol of the social outcast and can even by seen in popular women's magazines. But remember that these are permanent tattoos! And once you have one, it could be yours forever. Even with laser treatment, a dark tattoo may be hard to remove. The beautiful red rosebud on the breast will wither and fade with age; the dagger encircled with thorns will look like a dead bush with a rusty knife in twenty years. But for those of us still in love with the idea of a tattoo, the temporary tattoo is the perfect answer.

Temporary Tattoos

This is the way to go. Available in dozens of designs in color or black line drawings, temporary tattoos are fun, safe, and erotic. Sold in drugstores, beauty supply stores, fetish shops, through adult catalogues and on the Internet, they last three to five days on the skin with normal washing; less if you use oil or moisturizer or rub vigorously where it is applied. If you want to remove the tattoo sooner, oil or moisturizer on a washcloth will take it right off. And next time, you can put the tattoo somewhere else.

A new tattoo process has become popular, as popular as it once was in the days of Cleopatra on the Nile and the sirens along the Ganges and Indus Rivers. It is called henna tattooing, which has become very chic in California and is now catching on in South Florida. It's all the fun and excitement of a permanent tattoo without the commitment. Lasting five to six days and easily removed with soap and water, a natural henna is used to dye whorls and curlicues, or any other design or image you like, on the soles of the feet, the palms of the hands, and other body parts. Some, liking Lt. Dax's spots on the TV show *Deep Space Nine*, opt for her set of leopard spots down the back of the neck. Others remember the sexily spotted aliens in the movie-turned-tv-series *Alien Nation*.

Edge Play

This is Perverati territory. Edge play is erotic role-playing near or at the "edge" of a submissive's or even a dominant's limits. Sometimes called "resistance scenes" when enacted with a female top, these scenes work well for a strong bottom since a captive, even a strong, resourceful one, can be taken by force or by trickery. Millions of people fantasize about sexual acts that are nonconsensual. The outward appearance of putting up a fight, of saying "no" is what makes these scenes so incredibly hot. Often edge play fantasies live in the realm of fantasies that are nice to think about but don't really want to happen to us. But then one comes along and it just eats at you and eats at you and suddenly it is in the realm of the "maybe's" and shortly thereafter, it becomes a definite "yes."

Playing near the edge of nonconsensuality is hot and the closer to the edge you get, the hotter it becomes. It might be something that has an element of danger to it like being kidnaped and "gang-raped" or being given to someone as a sex toy for an hour, a night, or a specific service. Unlike "bathtub fantasies," (see Introduction) which are best left to the imagination, edge-play fantasies are something that can actually be arranged by a loving partner with no risk of physical danger. But this can raise emotional risks.

The emotional risk in edge play is the unknown factor. Suppose one of you has had a bad or very negative experience as a child.

Although you have thoroughly discussed the scene beforehand, something that was said or done in the scene has triggered old memories. You may not even know you have these memories but there they are. If you think there might be a problem with an aspect of a scene or the scene itself, you should bring it up before you start. I wouldn't want to be surprised by this kind of powerful emotion and neither would you. But it has happened and now you are a mess. What could trigger these memories? Just about anything, depending on who you are and what has happened to you. Some are freaked out by a slap in the face; others by a mere word said in a specific tone of voice or with special inflection.

Now what do you do? One of two things: You can stop the scene or play it through and see what is behind the strong emotion. Since you are new to this and there are powerful emotions in play, I would stop the scene and talk about it. Playing it through is emotionally risky for top and bottom alike. You may not be ready for this. So stop and get assurances that you will do this with him only if he is willing to work through some heavy emotional stuff. He needs to be supportive of you throughout the entire experience.

It takes courage to play on the edge. Always have a safe word to use in case real-world emotions arise and make sure you trust the person who takes you to the edge.

Electrotorture

Let's start by answering a basic question: who would want to have electricity applied to their body and why? Anyone of the Perverati could get a "charge" out of it and, aside from the pain and fear aspects, mild electrical stimulation of the genitals can produce intensely sexual sensations, even orgasm.

But make no mistake: Electrotorture is high-risk, dangerous play even by Perverati standards. *Electric shock can disrupt the rhythm of the heart, which can cause death.* Is there any part of that which is unclear? Good. Electric shock produces very intense pain, and there are other ways you can play with electricity that are much less painful and somewhat safer.

Electric Shock

Fantasies of electrotorture fall into two main areas: psychological and physical. Electric shock torture calls to mind any number of fascinating images from sadistic nurses to interrogations by the Gestapo or even the local police! Please understand that many who fantasize of electrotorture enjoy a good psychological trip. Set up the scene with all the appropriate accoutrement, your wardrobe included. Then apply something mild below the waist line. *(Never, never, never put anything above the waist!)* I have a little handheld face electromassager that feels nice in a tingly, staticy way and when he is blindfolded he has no idea at all what it is. Others have experimented with the weak shock from a nine-volt battery. This mild stimulation combined with the scene you have set up and what is happening in his mind can be a very intense experience.

The Violet Wand

If you want to play with electricity, this is how to do it! The easiest way to explain the violet wand is to compare it to the shock you get when you walk across a carpet. The shock can range from mild to wild and looks absolutely phenomenal. At a fetish weekend in Tampa, I borrowed one from a vendor and used a middle setting to relieve lower backache from platform shoes. I want one of these things.

A high-frequency circuit is used to build up the charge. Then a static charge is built up in the glass tube that is filled with gas. Although the shock is similar to that of a carpet, unlike shuffling across the room, the wand can deliver many sparks in a second. The unit comes with an on-off switch and a power control and is handheld. When switched on, the unit emits a sputtering, crackling noise which is quite fearsome to the submissive but actually totally harmless. Since there is no current, you can use the wand almost anywhere on the body except the eyes. *Never insert the glass tubes into any body openings.* Many models of the violet wand come with three attachments: a mushroom, rake, and tube. Sometimes, two sizes of mushrooms are available, a four- or two-inch diameter. The greater the surface area on the attachment, the weaker the charge.

Beautiful visuals can be made with the large mushroom. When I first saw the violet wand, the male dominant had touched it to the arm of his slave girl. She was outlined in an unearthly blue light, like a goddess of pain from another time and place shimmering inside her electric field, writhing in delight.

The tube attachment can be used to torture oh-so-many places on the male body with all its interesting protuberances! Wave the tube about half an inch from the end of his cock. He will scream as the stream of sparks jump across the gap but that will be before he realizes that on the proper low setting it hardly hurts at all!

Fisting

The invasive thrust of a hand entering your anus or your vagina is a provocative fantasy for many submissive men and women. For the Perverati it is a reality. On the physical level, the pain to be endured and the concentrated effort the receiver must make to assist in his own invasion make fisting an exotic fantasy. On an emotional level, the fist is a symbol of power, and working one into an anus carries tremendous impact and sexual charge. It may convey a sense of helplessness, humiliation, violation, and erotic submission. Fisting has a profound impact on its partners. Although the image of one person with a hand or arm deep inside the ass of another has mind-blowing dominant overtones, there are those for whom it is deeply spiritual, profoundly sensual, and even magical. As you move your hand in past the sphincters and rest it between them and the puborectal sling, it will feel like you are touching his soul.

As in all things D&S, fisting takes two, even though each partner will make separate preparations. For the top, nails must be short and smoothly filed even though latex gloves will be worn. All rings and other arm jewelry must be removed. For the bottom, two to three enemas may be necessary depending on the depth of play. The bottom will also need to train his muscles to accept larger and larger dildos until he can accept one that is at least three inches in diameter. If he can take a dildo that size, his anus is physically ready to take a hand. Additionally, the bottom must learn to control and relax his anal sphincters along with a host of other muscles that are normally under semiconscious control. Fisting does not necessarily entail great pain—that will depend on the ability of the receiver to relax and the giver to correctly read her partner's body.

And much depends on adequate lubrication. Remember! The anus and rectum are composed of delicate tissues and membranes that can be torn easily. *Nothing should ever be forced into the anus.* Condom lubricants like K-Y Jelly, Probe, and other water-based sex lubes are bad choices for anal fisting. They are thin and tend to dry out over the length of a fisting session. Crisco, yes, good old lard in the can, Crisco is still the number one choice among fisters. (Crisco is not good for intercourse with condoms.)

Do you want to know how to do this? Okay. Let's assume he has been stretching his anus and can accommodate a dildo that is at least three inches in diameter. He is emotionally prepared to have your hand inside of him. You have made your preparations and are emotionally prepared to enter him.

Let him assume a comfortable position, facedown with his hips over pillows or faceup with his hips raised. Position yourself and your supplies—lots of lube, gloves, paper or cloth towel between his legs. Lubricate your hand and arm generously and apply additional lubrication to the fistee's anus. The fister then inserts one finger, then two, in the anus. Work his muscle gently to loosen him, and when your partner's muscles seem relaxed the third finger is added. When the third finger is added, you should begin to fold your fingers under each other so they look like a triangle. Again, stroke your fingers in and out of him, loosening his muscle for the next phase. After he has taken the three fingers comfortably it is time to "restack" your hand.

Now your middle and ring finger should be on top with the pinkie and index fingers tucked under the top two and the thumb in between. This is called "the Swan" because it looks like the head and neck of one. As you slowly work your hand inside, there are several sphincters and valves that block your progression. These are opened by massaging or stretching the entrance area. An in-and-out twisting action can be started at this point then push one or two of your fingers through, gently pulling some of the intestinal wall down. Once the hand is inside him, move it around gently. The feeling is incredible since the hand is so much more dextrous than a dildo.

When you are ready to withdraw, remove the fist slowly to prevent the hand from creating a vacuum effect and pulling a section of the intestine out with it.

Pain is a definite indication of improper and dangerous manipulation. Since the anal wall is thin and could require surgery and the need to wear a colostomy bag if torn, proper fisting technique is essential. Fisting is not considered safe sex, but several associations in Chicago, Fort Lauderdale, San Francisco, and Washington, D.C., offer clubs for fisters where proper techniques can be learned in person.

Sexual Asphyxiation

Sexual asphyxiation is breath control as sex play. This is very dangerous and is best left in the realm of fantasy for all but the most experienced of the Perverati. Safe words do not work here because the sub won't be able to speak, and in general, this is scary stuff. I do not recommend that you undertake this activity under any circumstances.

In the playful category, many men like to be "smothered" and this is the most popular type of breath control, as it is the least risky. It usually involves something fun for him as well as air deprivation. For this play, you would sit on his face. I mean literally, usually with panties, for brief but increasing periods of time. In the fantasy, he has committed some infraction and this is to be his punishment. Alternatively, it is done to him to humiliate him and show him his place.

In this scenario, his first infraction earns him a count of "ten," as in ten seconds. For ten seconds you sit on his face and "smother" him, then get up. The next infraction earns a count of twelve or fifteen and so on, increasing his "punishment" by two- to five-second intervals each time. Of course, any male adult aware enough to play D&S games can hold his breath for ten or twenty seconds, or even thirty or sixty. Additionally, since you are wearing panties and your body doesn't totally smother his face, the risk factor becomes more manageable for a sensible and sensitive top. (And since he is much bigger and stronger than you, he can toss you off even though you are sitting on his face.)

It is vitally important before you start sitting on his face that the two of you discuss what his maximum "count" will be. Time it out on a stopwatch if you must, but do it.

The next most popular method of breath control is simple: Just clap your hand over his mouth, or tape it shut with a piece of low-density, three-inch-wide black electrical tape, then pinch his nose closed. Do one nostril, then the other, then both. *Always* look into his eyes as you do this. His eyes will tell you what is happening with him since he will not be able to speak. And his eyes can be his safe word. When he has had enough you could have him blink really hard or blink three times fast. But we are talking about a *blink*, something that is very easy to miss if you are blinking at the same time. A ball held in his hand to be dropped could be a signal, too, but again, this is risky stuff.

Sexual asphyxiation is mainly about control and fear. As we have said, fear is a strong aphrodisiac, and, in this play, both top and bottom will experience it. The dominant's fear will be timing and keeping the sub's fear at an erotic level. The sub will fear losing consciousness, or a "little death." *The play should NEVER go so far that the sub loses consciousness.* The control aspect for the dominant is tremendous. The fear in her partner's eyes as he thrashes about is an extraordinary turn-on as is the thrashing itself. For the submissive, the complete loss of control, the absolute trust in the top, and maybe even the light-headed, floating/drifting feeling is the turn-on.

Some recommend smothering the submissive with a plastic bag. Sorry, I find this horrifying. It is ugly to behold, unromantic, and positively frightening. It would be a very submissive sub indeed who would sit still while you put a plastic bag over his head. I would recommend that you stay away from this type of play and experiment with something that matches the beauty in your soul.

~ 18 ~

Prior Proper Planning

In the Introduction, I spoke of the Three P's of D&S: Prior Proper Planning. A very good idea, but possibly an intangible one if you are new to the scene, or simply don't know where to start. So I've laid out a general plan consisting of nine steps to help you conduct your first sexy and successful D&S playtime. Steps one, two, three, and four, which deal with negotiating and setting up the scene, should remain constant until you are more familiar with your partner's wants and desires and are more experienced at D&S. Steps five, six, and seven, the action steps, can be arranged in any order that suits you. Additionally, some of those steps can be considered optional according to your preferences or the particular scene. The eighth step, finishing the session, is standard but can be reworked to suit your taste. Step nine, cuddling and communication, is always important (and often the best part!) and should be considered a constant even after you have acquired some experience.

Your Playtime Checklist

1. *Talk it over.* You have discussed beforehand what you are going to do during playtime, what his favorites are, what his and your limits are, have chosen his safe word, and have made the necessary adjustments to accommodate both of you. Also, this is when you will decide how long your playtime will last.

2. *Create the right atmosphere.* Dim the lights. Get the music going and the candles lit. Make sure the room is warm enough and smells good. Incense will help here. Turn the answering machine on, and hope no visitors stop by.

Then, take time to prepare your mind and body for the upcoming experience. Your partner should also be preparing himself according to your instructions.

3. *Get your toys ready.* Put the objects you have decided to incorporate into your play someplace close at hand. These objects could include: collar and leash, piece of lace, nipple clamps or clothespins, makeup (for cross-dressers), handcuffs (and key!), blindfold or sleep mask, candles for waxing, scarves or rope and scissors, and a whip, or any other visible symbol of your authority. Make sure your safety gear is nearby, especially when playing at bondage.

4. *Step into your role.* Give him the signal that you are ready to begin by placing his collar around his neck, or the lace over his wrists, or by saying the phrase you have agreed to signal the start of playtime.

5. *Give him things to do.* Tell him what you want him to do for you. Assess his performance. Praise him when he deserves it. Make note of his mistakes and reinstruct him in your preferences. Tell him that he will be punished for unsatisfactory service—perhaps that will improve his memory and performance.

6. *Do things to him.* Pinch his nipples. Slap his breasts. Tie him up. Blindfold him. Whip him lightly. Slap his cock with the flat of your hand (gently, at first!). Then caress him and slap him again. Continue this action to start "conditioning" him. Try wrapping your hand around the base of his cock and squeezing. Then try doing the same squeezing action to his balls, building up slowly. Let go and begin again. Scratch him with your nails but not hard enough to break the skin.

7. *Dole out punishment.* If he has displeased you, or you just feel like giving him a beating, I find a beating at the end of the session to be the strongest sensation of all. If you are beating him to correct his mistakes, reiterate those mistakes and extract a promise of better service next time. If the beating is for your pleasure, tell him how much you enjoy beating him. Praise him for his acceptance of your will. Punishment or pleasure, I try to make the last ten strokes much harder

than any of the previous ones so that he will have to stretch to take them.

8. *Finish the session.* The grand finale of a session is usually orgasm for at least one of you. Have him perform cunnilingus on you, or present various parts of your body to him to worship. You could use this opportunity (I do!) to direct him in your idea of the proper execution of these services. Since you are still in your roles as mistress/slave the risk of offending him with these instructions is greatly reduced as he is still under your spell. After he has been rewarded, remove his collar or symbol of slavery with the same ceremony as you put it on. If you started by draping a piece of lace or ribbon over his wrists, end by redraping his wrists and as you take the lace off say something that has a ring of ritual to it, like: "I now free you from my service," or "I free this slave for his good service to me."

Now you are out of role. Climb on, grab a hold, make it a great event for both of you. Or you may chose to leave his symbol of submission on during the grand finale and continue to give him instruction in your role as mistress as how to please you more fully.

9. *Snuggle afterwards.* Cuddling and physical closeness are very important now. This has been a dramatic experience for both of you and you have different feelings about the experience. One or both of you may feel exhilarated, almost high; alternatively, you may feel a little sad or depressed or angry after the session. Playing with D&S is playing with strong emotions and sometimes old memories can come to the surface and cause distress. Talk this out; each will need reassuring that these feelings are not the fault of the other. Sometimes, a little extra time is needed for the feelings to be sorted out before discussion. Mention them then when you have come to a conclusion or decision, set aside some time to discuss these feelings when you won't be disturbed.

As you gain more experience in the art of sensual female domination and expand your "fantasy base," the likelihood of your slave becoming totally immersed in the fantasy and "going under" increases. After these scenes, he may seem a little befuddled or spaced or giddy. This is his body's natural response to the new sensations you have been giving him. He may be in a vulnerable state when you are through. Tell him how much you enjoyed playing with him, cuddle and nest and be sure to give him all the affection he needs as he returns to Planet Earth. Some scenes, even the playful, loving ones you will be enacting, can get very intense. This is good since it shows communication between you is open and free.

You may also be feeling a little vulnerable after your first session. For those of you not yet totally at ease with showing your dominant side, feelings of guilt and/or anxiety may emerge. Your partner should understand your need for affection and support at this time, just as you understood his. If he liked the D&S scene he shared with you, it is in his best interest to let you know how much he enjoyed and appreciated you! This supportiveness should be encouraged in the hope that it will carry over into your everyday lives and make them more pleasant and fulfilling for both of you.

I think you now understand the beauty and trust of the D&S relationship and are aware that communication is at its root. For several playtimes, you will still be flying with a net until you know what works for you. Pay attention to the person who has given you his body and mind and heart to "play" with as your "toy" and look upon it as the rare gift that it is. Good Luck!

In Closing

When you took your first step behind the veil that shrouded the "mysteries" of D&S, I am sure you had some reservations about what you would find. And although I did not want to strip my beloved S&M of its aura, I did want to make that aura easier to penetrate and more accessible to those seeking its power and sexuality. I believe that if S&M could ever be fully explained, and many have tried, it would lose its power to lure and seduce us. Like the vampires of romance, full exposure to the light would incinerate the dark beauty of consensual S&M. We need to keep it in our fantasy world; it needs the fertile soil only the dark side of the imagination and eros can provide; it needs its taboo to keep its appeal. Yet somehow we need to remove the stigma of "sick" from the world's overall perception of (even) erotic sadomasochism.

And as you finish this book, it is my hope that I have helped to contribute not to the "normalization" of S&M but rather to a more realistic understanding of the consensual D&S relationship.

Many members of the Perverati feel that, done with planning and the love of a caring partner, D&S can be a safe place to heal, change, and grow. Although each partner is strong enough to stand alone, they need each other for the acceptance all humans crave, for validation, for someone to trust with the erotic fantasies in their secret heart. As you play at D&S, never forget that you are holding your partner's trust and fantasies in your hand and extend around him the protective shield he needs at this time. Enjoy your time at the "top" but remember the one who put you there. What I have tried to present here is a combination of the basic psychological aspects and the basic physical skills and knowledge needed for an S&M lovestyle in a user-friendly format. I hope that as you finish this book one of the things you have come away with is a stronger sense of the personal power and eroticism you carry inside of you. That power is just waiting to be tapped into and let out.

And just in case I haven't said those two little words often enough, I'll say them one more time: "Communicate!" and "Practice! Practice! Practice!"

Appendix: Shopping Guide

UNITED STATES

California

Anonymous Leathers & Mfg., Ltd.
519 Castro St. #38
San Francisco, Calif. 94114
415-431-4555
anon@best.com
http://www.anonlthr.com
Custom leather, excellent whips, chain maille.

A Taste of Leather
336 6th St.
San Francisco, Calif. 94103
Catalog—leather, SM toys, magazines, custom work.

Adashi
1878 W. 11th St. #122
Tracy, Calif. 95376
800-832-2744
Fax: 209-836-0169
Dungeon equipment in stainless steel, custom fabrications, lubricant-safe nylon slings and suspension devices, chastity belts, wholesale/retail.

Black Eagle
8350 Santa Monica Blvd. West
Hollywood, Calif. 90069
213-650-9211
Fabulous leather creations.

Blowfish
2261 Market St. #264
San Francisco, Calif. 94114

415-864-0880
Fax: 415-864-1858
Very extensive line of audios, books, magazines, CDs, fetish fashions & equipment, jewelry, laser discs, and videos. Catalog available.

Bon-Vue Enterprises
901 W. Victoria, Unit G
Compton, Calif. 90220
800-827-3787
Fax: 213-631-0415
Excellent collection of BDSM and spanking videos; also, bondage art portfolios, books, photo sets, and magazines.

Bullock Leather and Accessories
7985 Santa Monica Blvd.
West Hollywood, Calif. 90046
213-665-5343
"Leather for Leathermen."

Butler's Uniforms
345 9th St.
San Francisco Calif. 94103
415-863-8119
Police uniforms and gear.

California Stan's
7505 Foothill
Tujunga, Calif. 91042
818-352-8735
Leather, lingerie, SM toys, adult toys, novelties, videos, CD ROMs.

Centurian
Vista Sta.

P.O. Box 51510
Sparks, Nev. 89435-1510
Mail Order/Catalogue
702-322-5119
"The largest fetish dealer in the world" has catalogs of "over 10,000 items" for all fetishes. One of the best.

Crypto Technologies Corp.
3132 Jefferson St.
San Diego, Calif. 92110
800-331-0442
Manufacturing and retailer (the Crypt) of SM gear, toys, books, magazines, and leather, owns 8 stores.

The Crypt on Washington
1515 Washington
San Diego, Calif. 92103
619-692-9499

The Crypt
1712 E. Broadway
Long Beach, Calif. 90802
310-983-6560

The Crypt at Wolf's, S.D.
3404 30th St.
San Diego, Calif. 92102
619-574-1579

The Crypt at Wolf's, L.B.
2020 E. Artesia
Long Beach, Calif. 90805
310-984-9474

Dark Garden
2215-R Market St.

Box 242N
San Francisco, Calif. 94114
415-522-9651
Beautiful, well-made custom
  corsets. New shop at:
321 Linden St.
San Francisco, Calif. 94102
415-431-7684

Draconian Leather by Metz
2325 Chester Lane #A
Bakersfield, Calif. 93304
805-631-8760
Free Brochure. Some of the finest
  handcrafted whips available.

Eastern Currents
3040 Childer Lane
Santa Cruz, Calif. 95062
800-946-9264
Needles and acupuncture
  supplies.

Erotec
6928 Shadowgrove St.
Tujunga, Calif. 91042
818-352-4344
Specialty toys including violet
  wands, erotic sculpture, SM
  toys.

Especially For Me
113 N. First Ave.
Upland, Calif. 91786
714-775-8356
SM toys, large bondage selection,
  lingerie, leather, latex boots
  and shoes; a Centurian store.

Fit To Be Tied
222 Main St. Suite D
Seal Beach, Calif. 90740
310-597-1234
Nice Latex, good selection.

Frederick's of Hollywood
Box 229
Hollywood, Calif. 90099-0164
818-993-3988
Lingerie, slutwear, you know!

Gauntlet
8720 Santa Monica Blvd.
Los Angeles, Calif. 94101

Piercing and piercing supplies,
  body modification magazines,
  videos, instructional materials.

Heartwood Whips of Passion
412 N. Coast Hwy. #210
Laguna Beach, Calif. 92651
714-376-9558
One of the finest crafters of
  floggers and cats in the
  business—and one very nice
  lady, too! Her catalogue is
  delightfully informative and
  highly commended.

Heartwood Corsets
412 N. Coast Hwy. #210
Laguna Beach, Calif. 92651
714-376-9558
Full torso corsets, custom made
  to client specification. I
  haven't seen these, but if her
  whips are any indication the
  quality is bound (no pun
  intended) to be superb.

Image Leather
2199 Market St.
San Francisco, Calif. 94114
415-621-7551
Custom leather and adult toys.

Iron Line
4001 San Leandro St. #30
Oakland, Calif. 94601
510-436-0662
Blacksmithing, collars, manacles.

JT Toys
4649 1/2 Russell Ave.
Los Angeles, Calif. 90027
800-755-8697
213-666-2121
Fax: 213-913-5976
tucker@oxy.edu.internet
Catalog—leather, sex toys,
  videos and SM gear.

Lashes by Sarah
415-621-6048
Excellent whips and floggers.

Leather for Lovers (Voyages catalog)
P.O. Box 77101

San Francisco, Calif. 94107
415-495-4932
415-495-5109
Mail order; leather and chain
  wear, devices and restraints;
  catalogs available.

Leather Masters
969 Park Ave.
San Jose, Calif. 95126
408-293-7660
408-293-7685
All kinds of fetish toys, novelties
  and fashions; catalog available.

Leather, Etc.
1201 Folsom St.
San Francisco, Calif. 94103
415-864-7558
415-864-7559
Manufacturers of leather, clothes,
  lingerie, and latex fetish wear.

Ledermeisters, Inc.
4470-107 Sunset Blvd.
Los Angeles, Calif. 90027
213-664-6422
Mail order: Male-oriented
  bondage gear, books.

Mind Candy Emporium
P.O. Box 931437
Cherokee Ave.
Hollywood, Calif. 90093
Catalog—rubber, PVC, and
  leather clothing.

Monique of Hollywood
P.O. Box 85151
Los Angeles, Calif. 90072
Lingerie, heels, boots, books,
  magazines, videos.

Mr S Leather Co. & Fetters USA
310 7th St.
San Francisco, Calif. 94103

also:
Mr S-2
4202 18th St.
San Francisco Calif.
415-863-7764 (voice)
800-746-7677 (orders)
Fax: 415-863-7798

Catalog—SM toys and bondage gear, incredible variety and a great reputation.

New Twist, Inc.
520 Washington Blvd.
Marina Del Rey, Calif. 90292
310-645-1069
310-645-3949
Manufacturing and distribution of women-only bondage videos.

Passion Flower
4 Yosemite Ave.
Oakland, Calif. 94611
510-601-7750
Fax: 510-658-9645
SM and other sex toys, leather, lingerie, books, magazines, videos, jewelry, music, etc. Female-oriented store and mail order.

Platinum Video
4501 Van Nuys Blvd.
Sherman Oaks, Calif. 91403
818-503-0280
Manufacutring of fetish videos and magazines, 150 titles, also sells equipment.

Playmates
6438 Hollywood Blvd.
Hollywood, Calif. 90028
213-464-7636
Lingerie, erotic fashions, PVC, latex, some SM toys.

QSM (Quality SM)
P.O. Box 880154
San Francisco, Calif. 94188
800-537-5815
qsm@cri.com
One of the largest SM and alternate sexuality literature sellers; also holds SM classes.

Rob of San Francisco
22 Shotwell
San Francisco, Calif. 94103
415-2582-1198
Catalog—SM toys and leathers.

Romantasy
199 Moulton St.
San Francisco, Calif. 94123
800-922-2281
415-673-3137
Sensual art and accessories for romantics, art, books, PVC, lingerie, Victorian corsets, jewelry, toys, soft-core videos. Catalog available.

Sarah's Bare Necessities
1909 Salvio St.
Concord, Calif. 94103
510-680-8445
Leather, SM toys, lingerie, swim wear, sexy outerwear for men and women, books, mags, hosiery, etc.

Seraglio
273 Milton Ave. (mail only)
San Bruno, Calif. 94066
415-952-6235
wander@hooked.net
High-end custom-made leather restraints and fetish clothing; specializing in unique corsets.

Stormy Leather
1158 Howard St
San Francisco, Calif. 94103
415-626-6783 (office)
415-626-1672 (store)
Excellent leather and SM toy boutique, leather latex, shoes and boots, bondage & SM toys, books and magazines.

Syren
7225 Beverly Boulevard
Los Angeles, Calif. 90036
213-936-6693
Rubber designs by Andy Wilkes (made Catwoman's outfit).

The Pleasure Chest
7733 Santa Monica
Santa Monica, Calif.
213-650-1022
800-75-DILDO

Catalog—one of the worlds's largest collections of adult sex toys.

Versatile Fashions
1040 N. Batavia
Suite C
Orange, Calif. 92867
714-847-5121
Manufacturing of B&D & fetish equipment, fashions and accessories. Also sells videos; 14 catalogs available.

Wayne's LeatheRack
4216 Melrose Ave.
Hollywood, Calif.
818-891-4228
Leathers, SM toys and custom clothing (located in Griff's Leather Bar).

Whiplash
3787 4th Ave.
San Diego, Calif. 92103
629-295-4322
Fax: 619-295-4301
Possibly the largest fetish store in California, maybe the U.S. Extensive line of Demask, Skin Two, Murray and Vern, Northbound Leather, shoes, boots, corsets, toys. A fetish emporium. Call for catalogue.

Xandria Leather Collection
P.O. Box 31039
San Francisco, Calif. 94131
415-468-3812
Fax: 415-468-3805
Mail order—fetish fashions and accessories.

Colorado

The Crypt
131 Broadway
Denver, Colo. 80203
303-733-3112
Large selection of SM toys, leather, books, and videos.

The Crypt Entertainment Center
139 Broadway
Denver, Colo. 80203
303-778-6584
SM toys, books, magazines,
  videos, and leather.

Dreams and Desires
1956 Wabash St.
Denver, Colo. 80220
303-329-0778
Lingerie, leather, lotions, and
  adult toys.

Imi jimi
609 East 13th Ave.
Denver, Colo. 80203
303-832-1823
Sensual leather.

Kitty's East
735 East Colfax Ave.
Denver, Colo. 80203
303-832-5155

Leather and Lace
2028 E. Colfax Ave.
Denver, Colo. 80206
303-333-4870
800-441-4695
Fax: 303-333-8141
Lingerie, leather, PVC and shoes.
  Catalog.

UZI
508 Colifax
Denver, Colo. 80203
Fetish rubber clothing and
  bondage gear.

Zip-Up Leathers
19 East Bayaud Ave.
Denver, Colo. 80209
303-733-7442
303-863-9233
Creates erotic leather apparel.
  Custom work available at the
  Denver retail store. Catalog.

Connecticut

Beth Tyler Labs
Box 2551

Hartford, Conn. 06146-2551
Fax: 203-871-0293
Interests are enemas, spanking,
  and bondage. Videos and
  equipment, also will shoot
  custom videos and photo sets.

Fantasy Isle
2 Mill Ridge Road
Danbury, Conn. 06811
203-743-1792
Adult & SM books, magazines,
  adult toys, SM toys and
  furniture.

Lacy Lady
530 Kings Highway Cutoff
Fairfield, Conn. 06430
203-259-7399
Lingerie, leather, SM and adult
  toys, books.

The Leather Harvest
1165 Main Street
East Hartford, Conn. 06108
860-290-8981
SM toys, books and leather, and
  those sexy black ropes in 50
  and 100 ft. lengths.

Rena's Ultra Boutique
76 Bank Street
Seymore, Conn. 06483
800-828-7362
Specialists in TV fashions and
  accessories, but have a wide
  selection of lingerie, bondage,
  leather, SM and adult toys.

Silk Stockings
68 Sugar Hollow Rd.
Danbury, Conn. 06810
203-778-5511
Lingerie, leather, SM and adult
  toys, videos.

The Water Hole
982 Main St.
East Hartford, Conn. 06108-
  2220
800-390-6674/860-528-6195
Fax: 860-528-3025
Brandrog@netcom.com

Custom leather and SM gear.

Florida

Christine's Lingerie
1124 N. 30th St.
Tampa, Fla. 33612
813-979-0154
Leather and lace lingerie, SM
  toys, magazines, videos,
  lingerie catalog.

Erotique
3109 45th St.
West Palm Beach, Fla. 33407
561-684-2302
561-684-2877
SM toys, leather, rubber and
  PVC clothes; books, and party
  info. Lovely store.

Exotique
Northwest Plaza
4023 W. Waters Ave.
Tampa, Fla. 33614
813-889-9447
Catalog—leather, rubber toys,
  and SM gear.

Fallen Angel
3045 N. Federal Hwy
Store 98 Coral Ctr.
Fort Lauderdale, Fla. 33301
954-563-5230
Catalog—SM toys, leather and
  gear.

Fantasy Island Innovations, Inc.
1304 SW 160th Ave.
Sunrise, Fla. 33326
800-785-9955
Mail order—leatherwear SM
  toys, books, novelties.

Fetish Factory
812 N. Federal Hwy.
Fort Lauderdale, Fla. 33304
954-432-0032
Fax: 954-462-6722
Specializing in latex and leather
  clothing from Europe, B&D
  accessories, magazines.

Glitzy Tartz of London
1251 Washington Ave.
Miami Beach, Fla. 33139
305-535-0068
Latex, PVC, corsets, shoes.

Leather Master
418-A Appelrouth Lane
Key West, Fla. 33040
305-292-5051
Mostly leather toys w/onsite
    leather workshop, but also
    sells rubber toys, erotic cards,
    magazines and SM books.

Metalbound Designs
612 NW 62nd Street
Miami, Fla. 33112
305-756-5245
Sculpture-like custom metal
    bondage equipment of
    unbelievable grace and beauty.

Outrageous Creations
PO Box 1608
Orlando, Fla. 32802
407-898-5897
Leather and rubber floggers,
    straps and paddles, hoods,
    harnesses, restraints and
    bondage equipment, and
    custom leather; lovely work!

Silk & Lace
8466 N. Lockwood Ridge
Sarasota, Fla. 34327
Lingerie, SM and fetish toys,
    adult toys, erotic fashions,
    private modeling services; ten
    stores in Florida.

Silk & Lace
1910, Suite A1, Courtney
Fort Meyers, Fla. 33903
813-275-6066 (see above)

Silver Anchor Enterprises, Inc.
P.O. Box 760
Crystal Springs, Fla. 33524-
    0760
800-848-7464
813-788-0147
Fax: 813-782-0180

Body jewelry (pierced) in
    surgical steel, niobium, and
    gold. Catalog.

Spice of Life Boutique
2940 SW 30th Ave. #2
Pembroke Park, Fla. 33009
954-458-5200
Fax: 954-457-8701
Sexy and fetish clothing mostly
    for women, books and videos,
    relaxed atmosphere, friendly
    staff.

Tender Moments
4635-3 Coronado Pkwy.
Cape Coral, Fla. 33904
941-945-1448
SM toys and books.

Underground Leather
1170 NE 34th Court
Fort Lauderdale, Fla. 33334
954-561-3977
Custom and ready-to-wear
    leather, BDSM gear and toys.
    Catalogue.

Georgia

Blast off Video
1133 Euclid Ave. NE
Atlanta, Ga.
404-681-0650
Kinky and cult videos.

LifeStyle Leather and Wood
156 Peidmont Ave.
Braselton, Ga. 30517
706-654-2702
Whips, collars, wood paddles,
    cuffs, clamps.

Midnight Blue
411 Cleveland Ave.
Atlanta, Ga. 30315
404-766-6288
Lingerie and leather.

The Pleasure Zone
1329 Brocket Rd.
Clarkston, Ga. 30021
770-414-1137

XTC leather, toys, lingerie.

Throb
1140 Euclid Ave.
Atlanta, Ga. 30307
404-522-0355
Latex, PVC, shoes, boots and
    accessories from top designers.

Warlords
2165 Cheshire Bridge Rd.
Atlanta, Ga. 30324
404-315-9000
Sensuous leather.

Hawaii

Submission
1667 Kapiolani Blvd.
Honolulu, Hawaii 96814
808-942-0670
Rubber, leather, PVC, erotic
    fashions, SM toys; also houses
    a piercing studio, "Paragon,"
    Body Piercing by Gus: 808-
    949-2800.

Iowa

Amazon Drygoods
Dept. H-6
2218 E. 11th St.
Davenport, Iowa 52803
319-322-6800
Catalog—corsets, historical
    reproduction clothing and
    patterns.

Illinois

C.A.T.
P.O. Box 25842
Chicago, Ill. 60625-0842
Corsets and dungeon furniture.

Dressed to Kill
3635 N. Broadway
Chicago, Ill. 60613
Fetish fashions.

Erotic Warehouse
1246 W. Randolph

Chicago, Ill. 60607
312-226-5222
SM toys, adult toys, books,
videos, mags, lingerie.

House of Whacks
515 N. Pulaski
Chicago, Ill. 60641
773-761-6969
Leather, fetish clothing, SM toys
and art.

Joe Wheeler
858 West Armitage
P.O. Box 104
Chicago, Ill. 60614
312-835-3468
Mr. Wheeler was apprenticed to
David Morgan. He makes
gorgeous kangaroo skin single
lash signal whips and other
whips with amazing quality at
reasonable prices.

The Leather Rose Gallery
1800 W. Cornelia St. Ste. 111
Chicago, Ill. 60657
312-665-2069
An all-in-one SM boutique, with
a lovely variety of SM toys,
literature and paraphernalia;
also has the Leather Rose BBS
312-665-0111.

Male Hide Leathers
2816 N. Lincoln
Chicago, Ill. 60657
Leather, rubber, boots, custom
work.

Paul C. Leather
2421 West Pratt
Suite 959
Chicago, Ill. 60645
1-800-FETISH-0
Gorgeous leather corsets and
fetish clothing at good prices.
By appt. only

S&L Sales Company
2208 N. Clybourn Ave.
Chicago, Ill. 60614
Fax: 708-963-2268

Mail order—resources, services,
and products for alternative
lifestylers; publisher of *Wild
Times.*

Silver Smoke
156-A E. Lake St. #101
Bloomingdale, Ill. 60108
SM toys, wood paddles.

Indiana

Naughty, But Nice
104 W. U.S. Highway 30
Michigan City, IN 46360
219-879-6363
Lingerie, fetish wear.

Kentucky

D.A.B.
1501 S. 7th St.
Louisville, Ky. 40208
Toys, books, videos, piercing
supplies, leather, and lingerie.

The Leatherhead Shop
1601 Bardstown Rd.
Louisville, Ky. 40208
Leathers.

Sun, Leather and Lace
1501 1/2 S. 7th Street
Louisville, Ky. 40208
502-634-4705
Tanning salon and leather
lingerie.

Louisiana

All That Jazz
419 Bourbon St.
New Orleans, La. 90130
504-522-5657
SM and adult shop with SM
toys, equipment and fashions,
books and mags.

Gay Mart
808 N. Rampart St.
New Orleans, La. 70116
504-523-5876

An adult and SM shop with
male emphasis, dungeon
facilities available for private
sessions.

Panda Bear
415 Bourbon St.
New Orleans, La. 70130
504-529-3953
SM and adult shop with a good
selection of SM toys,
equipment and fashions.

Rings of Desire, Inc.
1128 Decatur St.
New Orleans, La. 70116
504-524-6147
A beautifully appointed piercing
studio run by master piercer,
Elayne 'Angel' Binnie.

Second Skin Leather
521 Rue Saint Philip
New Orleans, La. 70116
504-561-8167
Excellent SM store; manufactures
own leather goods, very
creative designs; also
wholesales products.

Maryland

Firefly
3714 Eastern Ave.
Baltimore, Md. 21224
410-732-1232
Leather and lingerie, whips and
small equipment.

Indecent Exposure
14631 Baltimore Ave.
Laurel, Md. 20707
301-725-5683
Lingerie, video, and SM toys.

The Leather Underground
136 West Reed St.
Baltimore, Md. 21202
301-528-0991
Leather gear, clothes.

Montague Custom Leather
8954 River Island

Savage, Md. 20763
301-498-3398

Massachusetts

Eros
581a Tremont St.
Boston, Mass. 02118
617-425-0345
Top labels in fetish and parties.

Grand Opening
318 Harvard St. Suite 32
Brookline, Mass. 02146
617-731-2626
A women's fetish and sex shop with a great attitude. They have a dildo collection in an array of colors and styles that would make John Holmes hang his head in shame. Very female friendly.

Hubba Hubba
932 Mass Avenue
Cambridge, Mass. 02139
617-492-9082
Leather, SM toys, clothes, shoes, etc.

LJ Productions
1212 Boylston Street #192
Chestnut Hill, Mass. 02167
508-655-0337
Videos, paddles, and SM art.

*Marquis De Sade Emporium/Sickle
    Moon Creations*
73 Berkeley St.
Boston, Mass. 02116
617-426-2120
Leather and SM toys.

Toys of Eros
205 Commercial St.
Provincetown, Mass. 02657
508-487-4434
Fax: 508-487-4435

Michigan

Noir Leather
415 Main Street

Royal Oak, Mich. 48067
313-541-3979
Excellent selection of SM toys and leather fashions.
Also:
124 West 24th St.
Royal Oak, Mich. 48067
810-543-8733

Nevada

Erotica Plus
4029 W. Sahara
Las Vegas, Nev. 89102
702-362-0079
Lingerie, leather, lace, custom outfits, dancers' costumes, body jewelry.

Romantic Sensations
1065 S. Virginia St.
Reno, Nev. 89502
702-322-1884
10,000 sq. ft. filled with pervy stuff, including TV wear.

Unique Creations
3868 Pennwood #13
Las Vegas, Nev. 89102
702-365-1818
Leather and fetish wear, dungeon equipment, hardware, restraints.

New Jersey

Constance Enterprises
P.O. Box 43079
Upper Montclair, N.J. 07043
201-746-4200
Catalog—wide range of SM and fetish books, magazines and toys. "The Catalogue of Catalogues."

Dressing for Pleasure Showroom
590 Valley Road
Upper Montclair, N.J. 07043
201-746-5466
The retail store for Constance Enterprises has a wide selection of the finest quality

leathers, latex, shoes, boots, fantasy accessories and SM toys, each in separate showrooms.

Leather and Lust
424 Roselle St.
Linden, N.J. 07036
908-925-7110
Fetish and erotic clothing, spandex, leather, PVC, lingerie, whips and chains, bridal gowns, high fashion hosiery (including large sizes), and more.

Maspien Armors
67 Prentice Ave
South River, N.J. 08882
908-257-4890
908-254-6362
Leather and chain armor; their terrific "bearclaws" with workable claws still permit handling of whips.

Pleasurable Piercings
417 Lafayette Ave
Hawthorne, N.J. 07506
201-238-0305
Piercing studio and body jewelry suppliers.

Tim Swig Associates Group
Box 234
Stone Harbor, N.J. 08247
609-368-2482
Distributor for Posey and humane restraints.

New Mexico

George Hinson-Rider
300 Circle Drive
Santa Fe, N.M. 87501
Cane maker extraordinaire. Please write and include phone number or address for reply.

The Leather Shoppe
4217 Central, NE
Albuquerque, N.M. 87107

505-266-6690
Leather, SM bondage gear, adult
    toys and novelties.

New York

Adams Sensual Whips and Gillian's
    Toys
c/o The Utopian Network
P.O. Box 1146
New York, N.Y. 10156
212-686-5248 or
516-842-1711 (workshop)

The Baroness
244 East 3rd St.
#20832
New York, NY 10009
212-529-5964
Original latex designs for men
    and women.

Body Worship
112 East 7th St.
New York, N.Y. 10019
212-614-0124
Leather and fetish fashions.

Come Again
353 East 53rd St.
New York, N.Y. 10022
212-308-9394
Store is jammed with leathers,
    lingerie, corsets, videos, and
    the most complete book
    collection we have ever seen.
    Don't be put off by the
    salesmen. Catalog available.

Eve's Garden
119 W. 57th St.
Suite 420
New York, N.Y. 10019
800-848-3837
Cool womens' store with
    bondage gear, sex toys, and
    books.

Flesh Fetish
P.O. Box 7829
New York, N.Y. 10116-7829
CD of play music by brother and
    sister duo.

Gauntlet
144 Fifth Ave
New York, N.Y. 10003
212-229-0180
Piercing studio and jewelry.

Jeffrey's Toybox
521 Fifth Avenue
Suite 1740
New York, N.Y. 10017
212-989-3044

KW Enterprises
89 Fifth Avenue
New York, N.Y. 10003
212-727-2751
Mail order—bondage
    equipment, books, toys,
    videos, male-oriented.

Leather Lady
248 Rt. 25A
Suite 100-I
Setauket, N.Y. 11733
Catalog—leather, chain, and
    PVC fashions; standard and
    plus sizes.

Leatherman, The
111 Christopher Street
New York, N.Y. 10014
212-243-5339
Huge selection of leather and
    SM gear; helpful, friendly
    staff.

The London Boutique
84 Christopher Street
New York, N.Y. 10014
212-647-9195
212-206-0482 Fax
Extensive selection of leather
    and latex for women and
    men; custom tailor on
    premises, friendly staff headed
    by Andrea.

Lucifer's Armory
874 Broadway
P.O. Box 808
New York, N.Y. 10003
Bondage items, Sports Sheets
    and vampire gloves.

Nero Emporium, The
218 Plymouth St
Brooklyn, N.Y. 11201-1124
718-596-6376
Leather apparel & toys/medieval
    fantasy wear.

Pink Pussycat Boutique
349 Sixth Ave.
New York, N.Y. 10014
Leather, SM toys, and sex toys.

Purple Passion
242 West 16th St.
New York, N.Y. 10011
212-807-0486
Excellent selection of leather and
    latex for women and men, SM
    books and mags; helpful staff
    headed by Hilton.

Raven Distributors
25 Franklin St.
Rochester, N.Y. 14604
800-724-9670
716-262-2265
Mail order—Satin, leather, PVC &
    rubber lingerie, huge selection
    of nylons to sizes XXX
    (including nylons with seams
    and heel) also SM toys, clamps,
    restraints, fetish magazines and
    videos. $3.00 for catalog

Regalia
1521 State St.
Schenectady, N.Y. 12304
518-374-1900
Catalog—rubber, PVC, leather
    fetish fashions.

Rochester Custom Leathers
274 N. Goodman St.
Rochester, N.Y. 14607
716-442-2323

SAMCo - Home of SceneWear
    Originals
9728 3rd Ave. Box 514
Brooklyn, N.Y. 11209
718-748-7593
SM dungeon equipment and
    scene clothing, custom and

stock, private dungeon. Call for
appointment and directions.

Savage Leather
88 Central Ave.
Albany, N.Y. 12210
518-434-2324
Leather and toy store. Catalog
  available.

St. Michael's Emporium
156 East 2nd St.
Suite 1
New York, N.Y. 10009
Catalog—unique leathers,
  masks, collars, corsets, clothes
  and wonderfully made,
  unique leather armor.

The Noose
261 W. 19th St.
New York, N.Y. 10010
212-807-1789
Catalog—quality SM toys,
  leather, and custom work;
  newly expanded womens'
  wear department but not
  female friendly.

Venus Body Arts
199 E. 4th St.
New York, N.Y.
Piercing studio and jewelry.

North Carolina

Queen City Video & News
2320 Wilkinson Blvd.
Charlotte, N.C. 28208
704-344-9435
Books, CD ROMs, SM and fetish
  toys and fashions.

Ohio

Acme Leather and Toy Co.
326 E. 8th St.
Cincinnati, Ohio 45202-2217
513-621-4390
513-621-2668
Latex fashions for men, women,
  TVs, SM toys, videos.

Adult Toy & Gift
1410 Market St.
Youngstown, Ohio 44507
216-743-22051
SM toys, adult toys.

Body Language
3291 W. 115th St.
Cleveland, Ohio 44111
216-251-3330
Fax: 216-476-3825
Store for gay/les and SM,
  leather and rubber
  goods, books, magazines,
  videos.

Chain Link Addiction
13385 Madison Ave.
Lakewood, Ohio 44107
216-221-0014
Leather goods, SM toys and
  equipment.

Chain Link Addiction
11623 Euclid Ave.
Cleveland, Ohio 44101
216-421-7181
Leather goods, SM toys and
  equipment; also runs a
  piercing studio called Body
  work Productions in the same
  location.

Laws Leather
3016 Chatham Ave.
Cleveland, Ohio 44113
216-961-0939
Leather craftsman by
  appointment only.

VIPPS
P.O. Box 81508
Cleveland, Ohio 44181
216-899-1326
Portable erotic swing, self-
  supporting frame.

Oklahoma

Christie's Toy Box
1176 MacArthur
Oklahoma City, Okla. 73127
Adult and SM toys.

Oregon

The Blue Spot, All Adult Video
3232 NE 82nd
Portland. Oreg. 97232
503-251-8944
SM toys, large fetish and SM
  video selections, magazines,
  preview rooms.

Exclusively Adult
1166 South A St.
Springfield, Oreg. 97477
503-726-6969
Videos, SM toys, adult toys,
  lingerie.

Leather and Lace Lingerie
8327 SE Division
Portland, Oreg. 97266
503-774-8292
Leather, lingerie.

Spartacus Leather
1002 SE 8th Ave.
Portland, Oreg. 97214
800-666-2604
503-224-2604
Fax: 503-239-5681
Adult toys and leather goods.

The Leatherworks
2908 SE Belmont
Portland, Oreg. 97214
503-232-3280

Pennsylvania

Alpha Factor
Valley View Road
Box 6246
York, Penn. 17406-0246

Both Ways
203 S. 13th St.
Philadelphia, Pa. 19107
215-985-2344
800-429-7529
215-985-2020
Excellent SM shop, wide range
  of SM toys and leather
  creations, fetish wear, books,
  magazines and cards.

Danny's New Adam & Eve
133 S. 13th St.
Philadelphia, Pa. 10107
215-925-5041
Adult and SM toys, leather,
   videos, books, magazines.

Infinite Body Piercing, Inc.
626 South 4th St.
Philadelphia, Pa. 19147
215-862-3810
Http://WWW.lechatexotique.com
Nice variety of SM toys, books,
   etc.

Cindy Mohr & Liz "Tailor"
c/o Both Ways
203 S. 13th St.
Philadelphia, Pa. 19107
215-985-2344
Leather, corsetry, custom work,
   onsite expert craftwomen for
   Both Ways.

The Pleasure Chest
2019 Walnut St.
Philadelphia, Pa.
215-561-7480
Adult toys, novelties, SM and
   leather toys.

Zipperhead
South St.
Philadelphia, Pa.
215-928-1123
Large headshop with a lot of
   fetish fashions, some SM
   toys.

Rhode Island

Miko
45 Weybosset St.
Providence, R.I. 02903
401-421-6646
Latex, leather and accessories—
   even a fetish boat ride!

Sunli Specialties
221 Waterman St.
Providence, R.I. 02906
401-861-9258
Leather and rubber SM gear.

South Carolina

Bix E X-citing Emporium
4333 Fort Jackson Blvd.
Columbia, S.C. 29205
803-738-3703
Art, books, erotic and fetish
   fashions, SM toys, magazines,
   videos.

Chaser's Magazines 'n' Mixers
3128 Two Notch Rd.
Columbia, S.C. 29204
803-754-6672
Adult bookstore with SM toys
   and videos.

Texas

Chain Maille Fashions
1706 Norris Dr.
Austin, Tex. 78704-2808
800-729-4094
Catalog—metal fashions and
   custom work.

Christie's Toy Box
2614 SW Parkway
Wichita Falls, Tex. 76308
817-696-1851
Books, erotic and SM fashions,
   SM and adult toys, videos,
   magazines.

Christie's Toy Box
3012 Alte Mere
Fort Worth, Tex. 76116
817-224-8008
Books, erotic and SM fashions,
   SM and adult toys, videos,
   magazines.

Forbidden Fruit
512 Neches
Austin, Tex. 78701
512-478-8358
SM toys, leather, latex, lingerie,
   body jewelry, piercer on staff,
   adult toys and sex accessories,
   gifts.

Leather By Boots
711 Fairview

Houston, Tex. 77006
713-526-2668
Leather, PVC and SM gear.

Leather by Boots
4038 Cedar Springs Rd.
Dallas, Tex. 75219
214-528-3865
Leather, PVC and SM gear.

Shades of Grey
3928 Cedar Springs Rd.
Dallas, Tex. 75219
214-521-4739
SM equipment and toys, books,
   magazines.

Utah

Stocks and Bonds, Ltd.
P.O. Box 800-115
Midvale, Utah 84047
Complete line of bondage
   handcrafted equipment,
   custom work available; $5.00
   brochure.

Virginia

Fashion Fantasy
9013-A Centerville Rd (Rt.28)
Manassa, VA 22110
703-330-1900
Lingerie and leather toys.

*Giovanna & Silverwing Dungeon
   Designs (GSDD)*
P.O. Box 2423
Fairfax, VA 22031
703-515-HANG
Leather apparel, whips, custom-
   built dungeon equipment.

Night Dreams
8381 Leesburg Pike
Tysons Corner, VA
Leather.

Washington

The Cramp Leather
219 Broadway E.

Seattle, Wash. 98102
206-323-9245
Leather and SM toys.

The Crypt
1310 Union St.
Seattle, Wash.
206-325-3882
SM toys, leather, and videos.

Fantasy Unlimited
102 Pike St.
Seattle, Wash. 98101
206-682-0167
Large adult store, includes fetish
   fashions and SM toys.

Lover's Package
538 Rainer St.
Renton, Wash. 98055
206-271-9393
Adult shop, carries SM toys
   and fetish fashions. 12
   stores owned by PeeKay,
   Inc.

Lover's Package
2020 S. 320th St.
Federal Way, Wash. 98003
206-946-1061
Adult shop, carries SM toys and
   fetish fashions. 12 stores
   owned by PeeKay, Inc.

Lover's Package
401 SW 148th Payless
Seattle, Wash. 98166
206-246-6047
(see previous listing)

Lover's Package
3702 S. Fife St.
Tacoma, Wash. 98409
206-472-2584
(see previous listing)

Peekay, Inc.
901 W. Main A
Auburn, Wash. 98001-5222
206-351-5001
Fax: 206-351-0353
Owns the 12 Lover's Package
   stores. Handles and distributes
   all adult items.

Slimwear of America
P.O. Box 997
Eastsound, Wash. 98245
360-376-5213 or
800-892-4030
206-376-5213(voice/fax)
Catalog—latex fashion.

Toys in Babeland
711 East Pike
Seattle, Wash. 98122
Good selection of SM toys,
   books, and equipment.

Washington, D.C.

Dream Dresser
1042 Wisconsin Ave.
Georgetown
Washington, D.C. 20007
202-625-0373
800-96DREAM
202-625-2764
Leather wear, latex, lingerie,
   toys.
Catalog—Dream Dresser (mail
   order), P.O. Box 3787,
   Washington, D.C. 20007, 202-
   625-0377 Fax: 202-625-2761

Felise Leather
2613 P Street, NW (2nd Fl.)
Washington, D.C.
202-342-7163
Custom leather clothing.

The Leather Rack
Dupont Circle
1723 Connecticut Ave. NW
(2nd Fl.)
Washington, D.C. 20009
202-797-7401
Leather, rubber, and SM toys.

The Pleasure Place
1063 Wisconsin Ave., NW
Washington, D.C. 20007
205-333-8570
Novelties, adult toys, SM gear,
   lingerie, spandex, and vinyl.

The Pleasure Place
1710 Connecticut Ave., NW

Washington, D.C. 20009
202-483-3297
Novelties, adult toys, SM gear,
   lingerie, spandex, and vinyl.

Tiger Designs
1420 N Street, NW, #1011
Washington, D.C. 20005
202-232-8355
Custom-made leather and
   rubber restraints and
   harnesses.

Wicked Ways
Washington, D.C.
703-379-4735
wways@aol.com
Leather, toys, books; also
   sponsors scene events at "The
   Edge."

West Virginia

Market Street News
1437 Market St.
Wheeling, W.V. 26003
304-232-2414
Adult store, carries fetish
   fashions, adult toys, videos,
   etc.

Wisconsin

Naughty, But Nice
I-90 at Shopiere Rd.
Beloit, Wis.
608-362-9090
General adult and SM boutiques.

Naughty, But Nice
7070 South 27th St.
Oak Creek, Wis. 53154
414-761-9272
General adult and SM boutiques.

Naughty, But Nice
2727 S. 108th St.
West Allis, Wis. 63227
414-541-7788
General adult and SM boutiques.

Naughty, But Nice
W. 10521 Tritz Rd.

High 33 & 9094
Portage, Wis. 53901
608-742-8060
General adult and SM boutiques.

Tie Me Down
1419 E. Brady St.
Milwaukee, Wis.
414-272-3696

EUROPE

Belgium

Minuit
60 Galerie du Centre
1000 Brussels
Belgium
02-223-0914
Leather, plastic, rubber, high
  heels.

CANADA

Classic Shoe Co.
240-70 Shawville Blvd.
#76081
Calgary, Alberta, Canada T2Y
  2Z9
403-938-6491
Fetish shoes, stilettos and gear.

Il Bolero
6842 St. Hubert, 2nd Fl.
Montreal, Quebec H2S 276
514-270-6065
Latex, leather, PVC, monthly
  parties.

Northbound Leather
19 St. Nicholas St.
Toronto, Ontario
Canada
416-972-1037
Catalog—leather, latex wear, and
  SM toys of high quality and
  solid design.

ENGLAND

Ectomorph
Unit 1,

42-44 De Beauvoir Crescent
London N1 5SB
England
011 44 171 249-6311
Catalog—high quality fetish
  fashions in rubber, PU and
  leather.

Fetters
17a St. Albans Place
Islington Green
London N1 0NX
England
011 44 171-226-0665
Made-to-measure bondage gear.

Honour
86 Lower Marsh
Waterloo London SE1 7AB
England 011 44 171-401-8220
Catalog of rubber, PVC, shoes
  and bondage.

House of Harlot
Enquiries: 011 44 171 706-2315
Exclusive custom-made rubber
  fashions for men and women.
  Cleavage enhancement a
  specialty. Possibly the best
  designer of latex in the
  business.

Libidex
BCM Libidex
London WC 1N3XX
England
011 44 171-613-3329
Catalog—rubber fetish and
  bondage fashions.

The Magic Shoe Co.
Unit 6
88 Mile End Road
London E1 4U3N
England
011 44 171-791-3352
Catalogue: Latex knee and thigh-
  high boots, spike heels,
  stilettos, platforms, and
  commandos.

Marquis
P.O. Box 1426

Shepton Mallet BA4 6HH
England
011 44 171-831397
Makers of latex and vinyl clothes
  and accessories; 84-page
  rubber catalogue.

Murray & Vern
Retail Showroom:
20A Tower Workshops
Riley Rd.
London, SE13 3DG
England
011 44 171 394-1717
Pure collection in latex; Lycra
  and see-through garments.

Paradiso
41 Old Compton Street
London W1
England
011 44 171-287-2487
In Piccadilly; rubber, PVC, and
  lingerie. Fun and friendly.

Regulation
9-17 St. Albans Place
Islington Green,
London N1 9QH
England
011 44 171-226-0665
Catalog—military, medical,
  industrial, bondage, leather,
  and rubber. Great selection
  but very little in small sizes
  for women.

Skin Two Retail, Ltd.
23 Grand Union Centre
Kensal Rd.
London W10 5AX
England
011 44 171-968-9692 (voice)
011 44 171-980-8404 (fax)
Catalog—leather and rubber
  clothing to die for; high heels,
  wet look, corset, books, and
  accessories. Publishers of the
  infamous *Skin Two* magazine.

Voller's Mail Order, Ltd.
112 Kingston Rd. North End
Portsmouth PO2 7PB

England
011 44 1705 799030
Corset specialists, one of the big
  names in corsetry.

Westward Bound
Mail Order: 35 New St.
The Barbican
Plymouth, Devon PL1 2NA
England
011 44 1752 223330

FRANCE

Demonia
10 cite Joly
75011 Paris, France
43 57 09 93
Latex, PVC, and leather fashion,
  books, and body jewelry.

Phylea
61 rue Quincampoix

75004 Paris, France
1 42760180
French fetish and bondage shop;
  sexy catalogue.

GERMANY

Boutique Bizarre Reeperbahn
40
20395 Hamburg, Germany
040 317 5030
040 319 2060
The largest shop in northern
  Germany carrying latex,
  wet look, leather, corsets,
  high heels, magazines,
  books, videos and SM
  furniture.

Highlights
Gabelsbergerstr. 68
80333 Munchen, Germany

089 527475
Latex by Skin Two, Ectomorph
  and Murray and Vern;
  leather and PVC fashions,
  shoes.

<<O>> *Fashion Shop*
TECHCOM GmbH
Kronprinzensstr, 30
D-42566 Solingen, Germany
49-0202/56626
49-0212/549094(fax)
Fetish fashions.

THE NETHERLANDS

Demask
Zeedijk 64
1012 BA
Amsterdam, Holland
21 20-620-5603

Recommended Reading

Nonfiction

A Different Loving, Gloria G. Brame, William D. Brame, and Jon Jacobs (New York: Villard Books, 1995)

Anal Pleasure and Health, Jack Morin Ph.D. (San Francisco: YES Press\Down There Press, 1981)

The Anne Rice Reader, Katherine Ramsland (New York: Ballantine Books, 1997)

The Bottoming Book: Or, How to Get Terrible Things Done to You by Wonderful People, C. Liszt and D. Easton (available from Lady Green: 3739 Balboa Avenue, #195, San Francisco, CA 94121).

Dark Eros, Thomas Moore (Woodstock, Connecticut: Spring Publications, 1994)

Erotic Power, Gini Graham Scott Ph.D. (Secaucus, New Jersey: Citadel Press, 1997)

Figure Training Fundamentals, Versatile Fashions (Orange, California: 1997)

Learning the Ropes, Race Bannon (San Francisco: Daedalus Publishing, 1992)

The Loving Dominant, John Warren Ph.D (New York: Masquerade Books 1994)

Screw the Roses, Send Me the Thorns, Philip Miller and Molly Devon (Fairfield, Connecticut: Mystic Rose Books, 1995)

The Sexually Dominant Woman: A Workbook for Nervous Beginners, Lady Green (available from the author: 3739 Balboa Avenue, #195, San Francisco, CA 94121)

S&M 101: A Realistic Introduction, Jay Wiseman (available from the author: P.O. Box 1261, Berkeley, CA 94701)

Soul Mates, Thomas Moore (New York: HarperCollins, 1994)

Women on Top, Nancy Friday (New York: Pocket Books, 1991)

Fiction

The Ages of Lulu, Almudena Grandes; Sonia Sotto, trans. (New York: Grove Press, 1993)

The Amulet, Lisette Allen (London: Black Lace, 1995)

Beauty's Punishment, A. N. Roquelaure [Anne Rice] (New York: Plume Press, 1984)

Beauty's Release, A. N. Roquelaure [Anne Rice] (New York: Plume Press, 1985)

Belinda, Anne Rampling [Anne Rice] (New York: Jove Books, 1986)

The Captive Flesh, Cleo Cordell (London: Black Lace, 1993)

The Claiming of Sleeping Beauty, A. N. Roquelaure [Anne Rice] (New York: Plume Press, 1983)

Delta of Venus, Anais Nin (New York: Harcourt Brace, 1969)

Exit to Eden, Ann Rampling [Anne Rice](New York: Dell Publishing, 1985)

Jewel of Xanadu, Roxanne Carr (London: Black Lace, 1995)

Juliet Rising, Cleo Cordell (London: Black Lace, 1994)

Justine, Philosophies in the Bedroom and Other Writings, Marquis de Sade; Richard Seaver and Austryn Wainhouse, eds. (New York: Grove Press, 1965)

The Last Temptation of Christ, Nikos Kazantzakis (New York: Touchstone Books, 1960)

My Darling Dominatrix, Grant Antrews (New York: Rhinoceros Books, 1992)

Nine and a Half Weeks, Elizabeth MacNeill (New York: Dutton, 1978)

One Hundred and Twenty Days of Sodom, Marquis de Sade; Richard Seaver and Austryn Wainhouse eds. (New York: Grove Press, 1966)

The Story of "O", Pauline Reage (New York: Ballantine Books, 1973)

The Story of the Eye by Lord Auch, Georges Bataille; Joachim Neugroschel, trans. (San Francisco: City Lights Books)

The Whip Angels, Anonymous (London: Creation Books, 1995)

Venus in Furs, Leopold von Sacher-Masoch (New York: Blast Books, 1989)

Comic Books

"Lord Farris", nos. 1–4; "School for Submission", nos. 1–3; "Horny Biker Slut", nos. 1–10; and "The Bondage Fairies" (Seattle: EROS Comix)

Glossary

Anal play   sexual activity such as anal intercourse, rimming, and fisting.

"Bathtub fantasies"   fantasies that fall into the realm of really hot to think about but best left in the mind.

Bondage   any form of restraint applied to the body to restrict movement.

Bottom   submissive person in a relationship.

Cane   instrument made of rattan used for discipline or corporal punishment.

Cat o' nine tails   any multilashed flogger.

Cock-and-ball torture (CBT)   torture inflicted upon the genitals, including clamping, bondage, weights, clothespins, and cages.

Condition (v)   to develop a reflex or behavior pattern or to cause to become accustomed to. Much of D&S slave training relies on these techniques.

Corporal punishment   punishment inflicted directly on the body, such as whipping, caning, or spanking.

Cross-dresser   one who dresses in the clothes of the opposite gender.

Discipline   punishment or correction; or the training of a submissive.

Dominant, domina, dominatrix   female exercising authority or control, ruling, prevailing, the one who prefers to be on "top," in this case, you!

Domme   male version of the domina.

Edge play   role-play near the edge of submissive's or dominant's physical and/or psychological limits.

Electrotorture   the use of electrical stimuli to create a desired sensation.

Exhibitionism   act of publicly exposing parts of one's body that are conventionally covered, especially in seeking sexual gratification or stimulation.

Feminization   the act of making or becoming feminine, as in dressing up like a woman.

Fetish   any thing or activity to which one is irrationally devoted; any object, sexual or nonsexual, which excites erotic feelings.

Fetishism   condition in which erotic feelings are aroused by a nonsexual object.

Fetterati members of the second tier of D&Sers in the D&S hierarchy; rarely seen playing in public, this group attends club and scene parties for some titillation then go home to continue in private.

Fire & Ice the use of hot (as in wax) and cold (as in ice) for sexual stimulation.

Fisting inserting the entire hand into the anus (or the vagina).

Flogger any multilashed whip.

Flying, or floating rare and special transcendent state of consciousness achieved during a D&S scene.

Foot fetish sexual obsession for the feet or shoes.

Gag device placed in the mouth to stop or stifle vocal sounds.

Glitterati entry-level D&Sers; using D&S as a fashion statement.

Going under term describing a slave's emotional state when totally immersed in a fantasy (not as deep as *flying* or *floating*).

Golden shower urination on another person.

Head games domination where the focus is mostly mental, as in humiliation.

Humiliation playful humbling or teasing of a person about his desires, especially sexual ones.

Infantilism role-playing involving infantlike or babylike behavior including wearing and often soiling a diaper, eating baby food, etc.

Latex rubberlike material used in making tight, or restrictive, fetish clothing; often a fetish object in itself.

Leather mistress a domina who prefers to dress in leather.

Limits boundaries the dominant and submissive set for each other during the talk-it-over stage regarding do's and don'ts during the scene.

Masochist one who gets pleasure from physical or psychological pain, either inflicted by others or self-inflicted.

Master male dominant partner in a D&S relationship.

Mental bondage assuming a bondage position on command and "holding it" as if tied in ropes.

Mistress title of respect for the dominant woman in a D&S relationship.

Over-the-knee (OTK) classic spanking position.

Paddle a rigid, flat implement made of wood or leather used to smack a bottom.

Pain slut slang for a masochist who derives pleasure from physical pain.

Passable term describing a male cross-dresser who can fool people into thinking he is a woman.

Perverati members of the highest level of D&Sers; driven by their sexuality, these people are the entertainers of D&S and in a scene club, the dungeon mistresses/masters.

Playing engaging in a D&S scene or activity.

Player person participating in a D&S scene or activity.

Position training process of teaching the submissive to assume certain positions on command.

Power exchange empowerment of the female by the submissive's surrender of control to her.

Psychodrama very intense form of role-playing.

PVC (polyvinylchloride) shiny plastic used for fetish clothing.

Rimming slang term for engaging in anal-oral sex.

Role-playing enactment of a prearranged scene wherein the two players assume characters different from their own to better play out the fantasy.

Sadist one who gets sexual pleasure from mistreating others, or who gets pleasure from inflicting emotional or physical pain on others.

Safe word, or **signal** word or action used by the submissive to stop or slow down the action.

Sensory deprivation the taking away of one or more of the submissive's senses to heighten his awareness of the others.

Services the many things your sub can do for you.

Slave human being who, in a fantasy, is owned as property by another and is absolutely subject to her will; a person who is completely dominated by some outside influence, habit, or another person.

Slave training process of teaching a submissive to serve a dominant.

Spanking good old-fashioned hand-walloping delivered to the sub's bottom.

Spreader bar strong bar of wood, metal, or other material, with rings and cuffs attached to it to keep the sub's arms and/or legs apart.

Submissive (adj.) having a tendency to submit without resistance; docile.

Submissive (n.) someone who surrenders control to the dominant in a prearranged scene.

Switch change roles during the D&S session.

Topping from the bottom the taking control of a scene by the submissive person without attempting to preserve the illusion that the dom is in charge.

Transsexual person predisposed to identify with the opposite sex or one who has undergone surgery and hormone treatment to effect a change of sex.

Transvestite person who derives pleasure from dressing in the clothes of the opposite sex.

Vampire glove leather glove that has sharp metal tines or tacks lining the palms.

Vanilla sex term used by players for the sexual habits of non-D&S players.

Voyeur one who has an interest in viewing sexual objects or activities to obtain sexual excitement whether or not the other person knows of the viewing.

Water sports sex play involving enemas and golden showers.

Weights lead fishing weights or other weights hung from clamps, straps, or ropes that are attached to the body for torture.

Wrapping curling of a whip around a part of the body not intended to be hit.

With Thanks

Stepping Behind the Veil: Kevin J. McCain for "the Glitterati, the Fetterati, and the Perverati"

Bondage: Cynthia Lechan for the illustrations, Jennifer for Director's Chair bondage

Cross-Dressing: Brianna and Kimmie for makeup tips and mind set

Discipline: Janette Heartwood for her expertise on floggers, George Hinson-Rider for caning particulars, Cynthia Lechan for the anatomy illustrations

Foot Fetishes: Lindsay Moore for "The Pedicure," Cynthia Lechan for the anatomy illustrations

Humiliation and Head Games: Master Keith for pony boy/pony girl inspiration

Slaves and Slave Training: all of my sweet slaves for inspiration

Bits and Pieces: Kevin J. McCain for the title "Bits and Pieces," Jo-Jo Hughes for piercing information, Nona Sands for fisting facts, and Soft Sweet Mary for research

For her invaluable help, limitless patience and unwavering support: Lori Perkins, Perkins Literary Agents.

Index

225